"Today many personal trainers have forgotten what 'personal training' really means. After being an owner, director, fitness instructor, and personal trainer in numerous athletic clubs and fitness organizations for the past ten years, I have come to see many unfocused trainers using cookie-cutter approaches in their program designs. The result is "no result," along with frustration on the part of trainers and clients. This negative experience diminishes rapport and damages trainer/client relationships.

I applaud Ed Thornton's focus on improving trainers' listening skills and redirecting attention to the clients. If our goal is truly to help clients achieve a regular exercise habit, good listening can detect clues as to why clients may lack positive results. Listening creates a win-win situation.

It's More Than Just Making Them Sweat is a great resource of practical advice for trainers who want to start their own businesses or for those who want to improve existing practices. Ed's storytelling abilities and unique insights make his book easily understood by everyone wanting to succeed in these changing times. I am recommending this book to my colleagues."

—Nancy M. Kurzweil M.A.
Owner / Director of Prime Time Training LLC,
Continuing Education Provider, Personal Trainer, and Group
Exercise Instructor for the American Council on Exercise,
Post Rehab Specialist for The American Academy of
Health and Fitness Professionals,
Core Conditioning Consultant for the U.S. Olympic Ski Team,
Master Member of the International Dance
and Exercise Association, and
Master Member of the Reebok Alliance

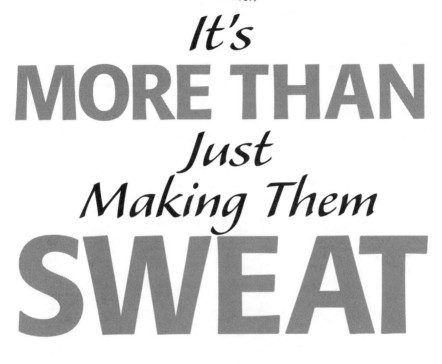

It's MORE THAN *Just Making Them* SWEAT

A Career Training Guide for Personal Fitness Trainers

by Ed Thornton

Robert D. Reed Publishers • San Francisco, California

Copyright © 2001 Ed Thornton

This book is sold with the understanding that the subject matter covered herein is of a general nature and does not constitute medical, legal, or other professional advice for any specific individual or situation. Readers planning to take action in any of the areas that this book describes should seek professional advice from their doctors, specialists, and other advisers, as would be prudent and advisable under their given circumstances.

Robert D. Reed Publishers
750 La Playa Street, Suite 647
San Francisco, CA 94121
Phone: 650/994-6570 • Fax: 650/994-6579
E-mail: 4bobreed@msn.com
http://www.rdrpublishers.com

Edited, designed and typeset by Katherine Hyde
Cover designed by Julia A. Gaskill at Graphics Plus

ISBN 1-885003-78-1

Library of Congress Card Number: 00-111629

Produced and Printed in the United States of America

to my parents,
George and Elena,
to my niece, Heather Lee,
and to all of my clients

Acknowledgments

This book would not have been possible without the painstaking assistance and patience of my personal editor and dear friend, Leslie Irvine, my word goddess.

Special thanks goes to Anne Thiessen, for her nutritional and dietary counsel, and to Covert Bailey, Barry Sears, and the instructors of the Boulder College of Massage Therapy, who have made otherwise dry metabolic and physiological science come alive for me.

I also thank Anthony Robbins, Napoleon Hill, Gangaji, and Dr. Wayne Dyer for inspiring me and encouraging me to have faith in myself through their meaningful work and books.

A special appreciation goes to Bob Reed, Pam Jacobs, and their publishing team for their expertise and guidance with the production of this book.

Last, and certainly not least, I offer my genuine thanks to my clients. Without their feedback, support, friendship, and willing bodies, this book would never have been written. Through the years, I have had the pleasure of associating with and serving some of the finest people I know. Not only have they given me the opportunity to learn how to run a successful business, but they have provided the insight I needed to become a more professional, more compassionate, and better person. You know who you are and I can't thank you enough.

—Ed Thornton

Contents

Introduction

A few years ago, a friend and I had a thoughtful discussion about the many lessons we had learned from our successes as well as our failures. After sharing our experiences, we both concluded that our failures had by far taught us our greatest lessons.

Now, although this revelation didn't come as any great surprise, it was still difficult to accept because it involved admitting that most of our working knowledge of finances, love, human nature, and spirituality had come through failure, and we had failed more often than we had succeeded in every one of those areas. What was even worse was acknowledging that we were the only ones responsible for our failures.

Trying to develop an appreciation for our failures, regardless of how much we had gained from them, was depressing at best. Yet, my friend and I found a certain comfort in knowing that we were at least in great company. We both could remember hearing "rags to riches" stories of people like Walt Disney and Henry Ford, who had failed repeatedly, losing everything, only to come back stronger and wiser each time they tried a new venture. Although the "failure route" wouldn't have been our first conscious choice for becoming successful, it did seem to be our best teacher, and, therefore, we had no other alternative but to reluctantly acknowledge it as a universal truth. In reality, we had much to be thankful for, because failure had given us some of our most valuable life skills, enabling us to survive, rebuild, and move forward after loss.

When the topic of success came up, however, we were forced to admit to being absolutely baffled by its nature, even though we had both recently begun to experience it in our professional lives. At that time, the only thing we had learned from success was that we really hadn't learned much about it at all, except that it seemed to be significantly more satisfying than failure. The more we recounted the thrill of being successful, the more difficult it became to explain why it was happening.

Within the previous year and a half, each of us had started separate businesses in Boulder, Colorado. I opened a private studio where I did personal training and nutritional counseling. My friend, being a chiropractor, finally opened his own office after sharing a suite in another doctor's clinic for four years. After a stressful and financially dismal first year, both businesses finally began to show reasonable profits, and, within the last six months, actually took on lives of their own.

As we considered other people we knew in our professions who were still struggling, my friend solidified our thoughts with this brilliant and eye-opening question: Why had we, of all people, begun to experience success at that particular time and place? In other words, why us? Why then? Why had the success that seemed so elusive just a year ago become so readily available now? Had we consciously shifted some paradigm, or were we just a couple of really lucky guys who took a leap of faith, and, after a year, ended up living in the land of gainful self-employment?

In spite of knowing that success had finally embraced us, we still couldn't help but feel vulnerable and frustrated, not knowing exactly what we had done differently to create it. All we knew was that we had both, very recently, become extremely busy doing exactly what we had always wanted to do: working for ourselves in our given professions. Granted, we had worked hard and paid our dues. But other professionals we knew had done the same thing for longer periods of time and weren't necessarily seeing the same kind of success. One thing we knew for certain was that out of all the chiropractors and personal trainers in Boulder, only a few found themselves so busy that they needed to refer their overflow clients to others in their field. The remainder couldn't seem to maintain enough clientele to sustain themselves financially. Ultimately, they were forced to find other, less gratifying means of support. After working for nine years as a trainer in different health clubs and recreation centers, I, personally, had witnessed roughly ninety percent of my coworkers looking into other careers within two years of starting. Although I was thrilled with my own success, it was distressing to think about the other trainers who were caught in the high turnover rate of my industry.

That conversation with my friend inspired me to look at the reasons why some personal trainers achieve success and others, no matter how honorable their intentions, don't. The book you are about to read will show you how to become one of the successful ones.

Let's begin by considering, for a moment, the majority of personal trainers in this country and why they may not be experiencing the kind of success they expected. Let's assume that most in this category are qualified, motivated, and in some way certified. Some may have degrees in exercise physiology, sports fitness, anatomy and/or kinesiology. The question is, why is this seemingly well-educated group of trainers sometimes unable to develop and maintain a clientele? Certainly, it's not their lack of qualifications. In theory, anyone with a legitimate certification or degree should be experiencing proportionately the same level of success in whatever area of the country he or she chooses to work. Why aren't they?

Let's now look at another group of personal trainers who **are** very successful. Although a lot of them share the same impressive academic credentials as the first group, interestingly enough, many don't. The truth is, some of the most successful trainers in the country merely sat through an eight-hour lecture, read a ninety-page manual, and then took a two-hour written exam to become certified. Did their lack of "formal education" hinder them? The answer is No! They are inundated with clients, they write books and magazine articles about exercise, and some have successful fitness shows on television. Many of these trainers, regardless of whether they work at health clubs or have their own fitness studios, are currently considered authorities on the subject of physical fitness.

How did they do it? Is there some mighty god of the fitness world that only bestows blessings of success on a few chosen trainers? Did these trainers find favor because they made a sacred trek to the Venice Beach

Athletic Club, where they sat in a special weight room and paid homage to the fitness god by diligently burning incense laced with protein powder on a Preacher bench altar? Or is something else going on?

What is their secret? What universal thread of success ties together the top trainers in this country? What distinguishing characteristics allow them to dominate the industry and command respect? The answers can be found in this obviously simple, yet profound statement: They see and think about things differently! Quite simply, successful trainers view the fitness industry through different eyes. Let me explain.

Top trainers tend to see our industry as a vibrant world, abundant with pure potential just waiting to be experienced. Their mission is to help people live longer, healthier, more active lives, and they embrace this as their calling. They understand the impact that exercise has in creating healthy physical changes in people's lives, and they love to witness these changes taking place.

In contrast, not-so-successful trainers lack this perspective. They see personal training in the same light as any other job in any number of saturated industries where most of the success has already been claimed by others. Some not-so-successful trainers look at their dwindling clientele and end up feeling jealous of the successful ones. They believe things like luck, geography, or great physiques were responsible for the others' success. They allow themselves to become disillusioned with this profession because they lack a consistent, weekly client base.

Perhaps the most important distinction between the two groups is this: when successful trainers go to work, they create an atmosphere of contagious motivation and achievement, wherever they ply their trade. When unmotivated, unsuccessful trainers go to work, they tend to get gobbled up in their own atmosphere of repetition and monotony. Those who have obtained degrees in some form or another often feel their education isn't being used to its fullest potential. Eventually, they leave to pursue other professions.

Because successful trainers unquestionably love what they do and, most importantly, **live** what they teach, they are able to inspire almost anyone with whom they interact. Whether it be in a crowded aerobics room or a one-on-one training session, they always exude a feeling of passion for health and fitness on top of being motivated, unstoppable professionals.

When the clients of successful trainers feel the impact of this powerful way of thinking, they can't help but get caught up in the vision their trainers have for them. This shared vision of achievement is what enables clients to believe they have the potential to do what they had thought was impossible. They are enthusiastically encouraged to achieve the impossible because their trainers can visualize them surpassing their accomplishments and know exactly how to guide them through their physical and mental transformation. The clients come away with the feeling that they, too, have the ability to accomplish anything they put their minds to, and this includes creating a new and healthy body for themselves.

Your Success in the Fitness Industry Starts Inside of You

It's More Than Just Making Them Sweat will give you the tools you need to see the results and experience the kind of success that our nation's busiest trainers already enjoy. My purpose in writing it was to offer a set of concrete, workable principles that you can integrate into your own fitness business through some very practical applications. Regardless of the level of success you may currently be experiencing, these principles will not only improve your business savvy and sharpen your training skills, but they will also increase the size of your clientele. What you will **not** find in this book are elusive, radical concepts that are out of your reach; rather, you will find easy-to-follow approaches that you can start incorporating immediately. These methods have been enormously helpful over the years in allowing me to help my clients surpass their goals, and I trust they will be equally helpful to you.

Whether you've been training people for ten years in your own gym or you were just certified last month and work at a recreation center or health club, this book will provide you with the information you'll need to establish the most successful fitness training business you can have. It addresses issues that could keep you from reaching your fullest potential and offers insights into your future training career. Much more than that, though, it challenges you to look inside yourself and take advantage of the opportunity to transform yourself into a more creative, compassionate, and knowledgeable person.

By doing this, you will gain a great deal. But it is your clients who become the biggest winners, because they will have been given new hope.

They will have a new approach to fitness with you as their coach. Together, you will develop a new understanding of their process, and the knowledge gained through this understanding will enable you both to tap the unlimited possibilities for mutual success. I believe that this new way of thinking is the foundation for success in the personal training business. Without it, success is fleeting for trainers and clients alike.

What Is It We Do?

Our job as personal trainers is obviously to assist people in making positive changes in their lives. How do we go about doing that? What are clients buying when they enlist our services? What makes them feel they're getting their money's worth? Why do some clients seem destined to fail and others make success seem almost effortless? What do we technically *do* for our clients and exactly who *are* we? The answers to these questions are quite simple.

People spend money to work one-on-one with a personal trainer for the purpose of achieving deep and lasting individual transformation. At one time or another, certain people reach a place in their lives where they need to change the way they've been feeling and living, due to any number of physical or emotional reasons. It is our job to guide them through these changes. In essence, what we become are guides to transformation. As guides, we must know where our clients want to go, how to get them there, and, most importantly, how to motivate them to stay focused on getting there. We must be able to visualize their success long before they do.

Certain abilities must be in place in order for trainers to reach this higher level of professionalism. These include:

🏃 *The ability to create a clear and concise plan of action that will enable our clients to reach their fitness goals.*

🏃 *The ability to lead our clients on a sometimes scary trek through, believe it or not, their physical identity.*

🏃 *The ability to communicate the importance of commitment clearly and effectively, so that when clients are tempted by inactivity or unhealthy indulgences they will not give in.*

🏃 *The ability to truly care about the well-being of our clients.*

🏃 *The knowledge and ability to back up our caring with action and results.*

🏃 *The understanding and mastery of certain principles associated with psychology, creativity, and communication as well as physiology, anatomy, and kinesiology.*

The certification you received upon becoming a personal trainer did nothing more than test your knowledge of the physical body, basic metabolism, and rudimentary training skills. These are all very important things to know; nevertheless, the way in which you **apply** that knowledge when creating your own system of training will determine your success. Your research, observations, knowledge, and experience mean nothing if you lack the ability to transfer them to your clients through a system of fitness training that is effective and uniquely your own. Your system must combine scientifically proven methods with savvy interpersonal skills.

In order to begin to create this kind of system, you must be able to say yes to the following three questions:

Question #1: Do you honestly believe that exercise and a balanced diet will cure or prevent most of the physical ailments of our human condition?

Question #2: Have you learned about and incorporated some of the best ways of exercising, eating, thinking, and living into your own life? (In other words, do you strive to maintain a healthy mind and body?)

Question #3: Do you love motivating others?

If you answered yes to these three questions, then you have what it takes to develop a successful personal training business. Why? Because you already are the type of powerful resource I've described, and clients will be more than happy to pay you for your talents.

But you'll get more than income out of this partnership. More than a thriving, lucrative business, you will enjoy the enormous gratification that can only come from helping other people improve their quality of life. Your role in helping each client do so begins with knowing why they may have failed in the past and then offering them the antidote to failure. This is what I consider to be one of the nicest perks of this business: that I can actually have a powerful impact on the lives and health of my clients based on my ability to help them succeed.

This possibility is what thousands of people across the country are spending millions of dollars on every year. They spend this money in our industry as well as many other therapy industries because they feel the need to gain control over some aspect of their lives that has most likely been out of control for years. By the time we see them, they're often discouraged, frustrated, and sometimes a little embarrassed because they've finally had to admit that, without a healthy and strong body, they can't fully enjoy any of the other successes they may have accomplished in their lives.

Why Listen to Me?

The question you may now be asking yourself is: What qualifies this guy to offer me all this advice on the business of personal training?

Quite simply, it is the fact that at one point many years ago, I was a complete failure at it, but at present, I have a business that is experiencing a very comfortable success.

In the beginning of my career, despite the fact that I acquired certification, studied the latest techniques in fitness instruction, attended the hottest seminars and lectures, and generally thought I possessed enough technical knowledge about human anatomy to fill a space shuttle, I still found myself failing as a personal trainer. Just one of the ways I failed was that I didn't realize the importance of combining my technical knowledge with an understanding of the different aspects of human nature. Another way to fail, I discovered, was by not really listening to my clients because I was too busy listening to myself.

Only when I realized how to balance technical knowledge with sensitivity did I begin to see the positive results of my endeavor in the form of a rapidly growing clientele. My knowledge of anatomy, physiology, kinesiology, metabolism, target heart rates, blood pressure, body composition testing, and exercise programs, in general, although extremely important, was just not enough to make people feel compelled to train with me week after week. It required the development of patience, understanding, compassion, organization, and boundaries to really make my business come alive.

As I've mentioned before, we who have been inspired to work in this profession do so primarily because of our love for fitness and our desire to help people reach their fitness goals. In spite of all our good intentions, we cannot lose sight of the fact that we are not just training bodies, but also working with egos, self-images, insecurities, and different aspects of self-esteem. Working with emotions as well as helping people experience the miracle of physical transformation requires being everything from a motivating partner to a therapist, a teacher, and a friend. We constantly walk the line between business and friendship, between involvement and detachment, and between success and failure. We are the guides who lead our clients through their sometimes rough and always challenging journey to the land of better health. This book is about making you a better guide.

In this book, I cover topics such as:

- *educating your clients about their bodies without confusing them;*

- *customizing exercise programs to fit your clients' individual lifestyles;*

- *establishing the kind of relationship that will ensure repeated business;*

- *knowing what people look for when they shop for a personal trainer;*

- *marketing your business and understanding the difference between prospects, customers, and clients;*

- *developing your creativity and not allowing yourself to become a "cookie cutter" trainer.*

If you have a working knowledge of anatomy, physiology, kinesiology, and a basic understanding of fitness training coupled with a sincere desire to be more successful in this field, *It's More Than Just Making Them Sweat* is your next logical step to mastery and success. I owe my success entirely to the principles found in the following pages, and I offer them to you in the hope that you will learn from my mistakes. Remember that the less time you spend in trial and error, the more time you can spend helping your clients get healthy.

Read on and greatly enhance your professional life. Happy training!

1 *Your Clients' Success Comes First*

My Two-Year Lapse

How do you define success? What will it take to reach it? In this chapter, I'm going to challenge the way you think about success. The three lessons I offer here will not only save you time and money, they will also spare you a lot of frustration and disappointment.

With that in mind, I'd like to begin by sharing some advice I was given a few years ago by a highly successful and respected personal trainer who lived in my town. Before I impart to you these gems of wisdom, I must confess that at the time they were given to me I was so lacking in good sense that I cast them aside with little regard for their importance.

Why didn't I take the advice I was given that day? The reason, I'm embarrassed to say, is that doing so would have forced me to rethink (and rewrite) sections of a business plan I had just completed, and it just would have been too much trouble!

The purpose in writing the plan was, ultimately, to establish an independent fitness studio where people could have the option of training with me on an individual basis, without the need to become a member of a health club or recreation center. As far as I was concerned, every minute detail of my strategy had been researched, organized, and finalized, including the way I believed I should think, speak, and act in relation to the work I'd be doing with my future clients. I had spent a full four months researching everything from where potential clients lived and what their income level was to how much of that income was spent on health and fitness and how happy they were with the results they were getting. The last thing I thought I needed was anyone, no matter how successful and established he was, telling me I may have missed something. Oh, the ego, in all its glory!

The time I wasted, the clients I let slip away, the money I failed to make, and the personal satisfaction I didn't receive were all part of the price I paid for not taking some simple advice that was freely given to me. Out of frustration, I even considered leaving what turned out to be the most rewarding profession of my life: that of a personal trainer. Don't let this happen to you.

Lesson One: Put Your Clients' Success Before Your Own
The advice I cast aside that day went something like this:

"Ed, don't believe for one minute that you'll ever become truly successful as a personal trainer if your own success is what you consistently focus on. Whether you choose to do your training in your own private studio or a large corporate health club, your talents and awareness must always be geared toward making the people you train successful first. If you concentrate your energies anywhere but on their success, you'll ultimately do it at the expense of your own success, because you will never be any more successful than your clients are. Just remember: 'You don't get to feel it or claim it until your clients first become it!'"

"That's it?" I said. "That's the most important advice you can give me about being a successful personal trainer? What about exercise programs, technique, skill, and personality, you know, all of the things that have made you successful?"

"Ed, my feeling is, you already have those things, and although they are very important, you must know that, in and of themselves, they cannot guarantee your success. The reason you stand a better-than-average chance of failing in this business is not that you lack personality, technique, skill, or the ability to create exercise programs for people. The reason I think you're going to fail is that all you ever talk about is how big and successful you plan to be!"

"What's wrong with that?" I asked in amazement.

"If you go into this field without the intention of seeing your clients' success come before your own, you'll be destined to become just another train wreck on the railway of well-intentioned entrepreneurial dreamers. And the first casualty of your ego will probably be that little fitness studio you've been telling me you want to start in the next few months."

Well, that certainly got my attention. But still, I chose not to take his words to heart, in part because I was already feeling successful just finishing my business plan! My logical mind wouldn't allow me to believe that such simple advice could be responsible for the incredible success I saw this man experiencing. A small part of me even believed that he was withholding his really important secrets for fear I'd become his major competition.

In any event, I ignored his advice, and struggled to make a living as a personal trainer for about two years. Then, as fate would have it, I came smack up against the same advice again. This time, it was an instructor at a fitness seminar in Denver who said more or less the same thing. After hearing the same advice for the second time, and having the benefit of some experience in the field, I was not only able to appreciate the practical wisdom of what had been said, but could finally see the importance of directly applying it to my struggling business. It was like finding the missing piece of a puzzle I'd been working on for the previous two years. I found myself saying, "Oh yes, of course! I knew that!" To this day, the fact that I was less than successful for the first few years of my career simply because I chose not to believe in and apply a principle that would have been so easy to incorporate still baffles me.

The way I saw it back then, taking the advice would have meant **thinking differently,** and that would have been an affront to my intelligence and perhaps even a threat to my manhood. (I was such an enlightened visionary!)

Please try to remember that although we often pridefully think of our ideas and business plans as being touched by the very hand of God, and we all know that words of advice are worth less than a dime a dozen, sometimes, it pays to swallow our pride, take the advice, and be willing to change our sacred plans.

Step one on the journey to becoming a successful personal trainer is putting your clients' success before your own. My assumption is that you want to experience true success as a personal trainer, and my hope is that you will show more wisdom than I by taking this advice to heart and using it as the very foundation of your business—or future business—today. It truly is the first step to any success you will have in this field, and without it you will struggle unnecessarily, as I did.

With this piece of the puzzle firmly in place, let's continue the journey to your success as a personal trainer.

Lesson Two: **Success Breeds Success**
Become a Partner in Health

If the first step to creating a successful personal training business begins with you placing your client's success before yours, then what comes next? The second step is to develop that thought into the ability to establish a positive, healing relationship with your clients, so that they always feel you are their partner in greater health and vitality. Creating this partnership is crucial to the success of your business because out of it grows the effort, commitment, and trust your clients must have in order to reach their goals. When this type of alliance occurs, it is akin to having a qualified, trusted family friend do your taxes instead of some stranger in a strip mall. Obviously, there is a certain risk either way, but the odds are you will have better luck working with someone you know and believe in, as opposed to someone who just finished number-crunching fifty other tax returns before yours.

Without question, a certain degree of respect and faith must be in place in order to develop this type of trust, but much more than that, you must establish the mutual understanding that you have what it takes to turn your clients into **winners.** This is what you bring to the partnership.

What your clients bring is their commitment to do the work and to pay you for your knowledge, time, system, and experience. Any doubts they may have about your abilities or their commitment are like huge cracks in the foundation of a house. Your clients may like, respect, and have faith in you, but the bottom line is that if you lack the ability to **deliver them to success,** they won't be your clients for long. Since your personal reputation as well as the success of your business hinges upon the success of your clients, getting them to see and feel the results of your program must become your highest priority.

So, what do I mean by "delivering clients to success"? In order to answer this question, let's look at some research that provides a better understanding of why some people become successful and others don't.

Every study or theory I've ever read has first stressed the importance of a person's attitude or state of mind in the attainment of success, and then offered some method to achieve it. Hundreds of studies have been done on the interaction between mindset and success. There are dozens of books written by consultants and therapists on how to apply these methods. It would take years to read them all. Fortunately for you, I've done some of that reading already. I'll tell you about the studies that have helped me instill my clients with a feeling of hope that they can triumph in reaching their fitness goals.

The process referred to as the "Matthew Effect" first appeared in the journal *Science* and helped form the basis for numerous books on education and psychology. As a principle, it has actually been around for about two thousand years, but the first comprehensive study of the process was done by a sociologist named Robert K. Merton in the late 1960s. It was based on a biblical passage from the Book of Matthew (13:12) that goes like this: "For whoever has, to him more will be given, and he will have abundance; but whoever does not have, even what he has will be taken away from him." Boy, it seems the "have nots" have always had it rough!

One of the things Merton did was to study the early and later lives of a large number of successful as well as unsuccessful individuals. What he found, with few exceptions, was that if a person experiences any kind of success early in life, he or she is more apt to encounter successful opportunities and environments throughout the rest of his or her life. The child's parents offer praise for doing things right. They set clear and specific goals for the child. Educators and mentors pick up where the parents leave off. Children who receive this kind of treatment are encouraged to accomplish their cherished dreams and make a sustained effort toward success. Along the way, they enjoy the camaraderie of other successful people who are headed in the same direction. They usually end up getting more of whatever it is they're going for in life, and that becomes the norm. Experiencing a lifestyle of fulfillment is what they come to expect, and the universe seems to honor their expectations. Recent studies continue to drive this point home. Psychologist Daniel Goleman's bestselling book, *Emotional Intelligence*, argues that emotional skills of the sort I just mentioned may be even more important than IQ when it comes to success and satisfaction.

In contrast, people who may not have received adequate nurturing and encouragement as children grow into adults who can't see the positive opportunities directly in front of them. They grow up unaware of how to seek out, get along with, and enjoy the company of other positive-minded, successful people, and they often feel more comfortable in the company of less-than-positive thinkers. Although they may feel comfortable in their misery, they never really experience true satisfaction in their lives because of the underlying envy and desire to have the things that the positive-minded people have. The result is they often lose whatever they have, including the opportunity to have a fulfilling and successful life.

What I'd like to stress is that the acceptance of either of these attitudes will have a dynamic effect on how we live our lives, because they become self-fulfilling prophecies: they create experiences that reinforce each other over time. (In other words, "The rich get richer and the poor get poorer.")

In the world of fitness, overweight, out-of-shape people tend to get fatter and more out of shape every time they finish doing the latest fad diet or exercise routine. They get more disillusioned, frustrated, and cynical with each new effort. They eventually fall victim to the false belief that their bodies actually lack the ability to respond positively to healthy stimuli. When they exercise, they often hurt themselves by overdoing it, in a subconscious effort to prove to themselves and others that they can't change. They get hooked into trying any new diet, pill, or electric abdominal stimulator that comes on the market, only to experience more failure, vulnerability, and disillusionment. At a certain point, they simply give up and stop trying. They often suffer premature deaths from heart attacks, adult-onset diabetes, certain cancers, or any number of other fat-related, preventable diseases.

Now, on the happier side: That same type of person, committed to a sensible diet and steady routine of the right type of exercise designed and monitored by a competent trainer, will experience small successes at first. These will be followed by larger successes, followed by lifestyle changes that lead to better health, increased longevity, and greater peace of mind.

The Matthew Effect is a metaphor for the level of comfort that each group reaches, and it is within that level of comfort—or comfortable misery—that our clients and we as trainers experience either success or failure. Even without direct knowledge of this effect, successful personal trainers subconsciously apply its simple truths on a daily basis. They get their clients to feel comfortable in the process of achieving their immediate physical goals and help them to map out their own long-term plans for fitness, health, and well-being. They assist their clients in developing a pattern of reaching these goals by using a system of exercise that allows each individual to take responsibility for and control of his or her own physical destiny.

Successful trainers also realize that the most current beliefs about the "best" ways to exercise and eat will inevitably change if one stays in the fitness industry long enough. How many times in the last fifteen years have carbohydrates gone from being "good for you," to "really bad for you," to "okay, in moderation," to, at the time of this writing, "good for you—as long as you do lots of aerobics and don't eat them in the form of bagels or pasta"? How many times, in just the last six years, has everyone from movie stars to plastic surgeons to football trainers to Navy SEALS not only discovered the newest ways to diet and exercise, but also felt the need to share their expert opinions on these topics with the rest of us?

Successful personal trainers live the Matthew Effect because they understand that the most important service they can offer people is to inspire them to build progressively upon their own physical successes by continually exercising in some form or another for the rest of their lives, regardless of what trends or diets happen to be in vogue at the time. They help people establish a subconscious motivation to stay physically active, in the same way they may feel motivated to take a shower or brush their teeth in the morning. When you can help people to develop the mindset of maintaining healthy physical habits over a lifetime, regardless of the different trends that will inevitably come and go, therein lies the success of your business, and your personal success as well.

I've never met a successful person in any field who didn't have a comfortable aptitude for achievement, as well as a healthy sense of self and a desire to help others become successful. This doesn't mean their lives are devoid of tension or strife. It simply means that, all in all, they feel relatively happy with the place they've made for themselves in the world, and out of that feeling comes the capacity to visualize future success for themselves and others.

The wonderful thing about playing with success is that it is not entirely necessary to have been nurtured as children in order to experience it as adults. Deep inside all of us lies the mechanism that enables us to start the process of becoming successful at any time throughout our lives. To be sure, when it comes to their bodies, people don't always believe they can do it on their own, and this is where some of their biggest frustrations lie. This is also the place in their lives where you, as their personal trainer and partner in health, can have the biggest impact.

The way this translates to your training business is simple. You must first have a comfortable sense of achieving physical as well as other types of success in your own life if you wish to convince your clients that they have what it takes to build it into their lives. Once they believe that it's possible, you must then make the process safe, comfortable, effective, and, above all, pleasurable. Without these four elements, your clients will most likely drop out of your program before seeing their desired results.

Lesson Three: Cultivate Pleasure and Flow States

An important part of the process of achieving physical success involves making it a pleasurable experience. The reason people stop exercising is that it becomes boring and unpleasant. So let's look at what motivates this need for pleasure and consider how we can use it to guide our clients in their journey to better health.

Human beings perpetually seek pleasure, in some form or another, starting at birth and continuing throughout our lives. Since most of us know all too well the problems that can arise when we seek pleasure in less-than-healthy forms, the trick is to skillfully cultivate an appreciation for pleasures that will not harm us and can even be good for us.

The problem that frequently comes up for personal trainers is that some clients, even after making great strides and reaching many goals, have the tendency to backslide into the same old habits or negative pleasures that got them into trouble in the first place. This could be anything from overeating, to not exercising, to smoking, to living on their couches.

In order to motivate our clients to keep reaching for and achieving their physical goals, we must first help them to recognize, appreciate, and gravitate toward the positive side of Pleasureland. This task may involve inspiring them to undo as many as thirty years of junk food and physical laziness. This is where your logic, reason, and motivational skills become invaluable.

A little understanding of how the human race developed the need to seek pleasure, both healthy and unhealthy, can greatly enhance your ability to keep your clients pointed in the right direction.

Many behavioral scientists have studied the human need to seek pleasurable experiences. For our purposes as trainers, I want to focus on one in particular. His name is Mihaly Csikszentmihalyi (pronounced Muh-hi Chick-sent-muh-hi), and he is a professor of psychology at the University of Chicago. He coined the psychological term "flow," and his writings have helped millions of people understand what motivates, stimulates, and inspires individuals to do their best at whatever they are pursuing. After reading the research outlined in Csikszentmihalyi's best-selling book, *Flow: The Psychology of Optimal Experience,* a *New York Times Book Review* critic had this to say: "Flow is important. . . . The way to happiness lies not in mindless hedonism, but in mindful challenge."

Csikszentmihalyi defines flow as an optimal experience, "those times when people report feelings of concentration and deep enjoyment." He writes:

> Contrary to what we usually believe, moments like these, the best moments in our lives, are not the passive, receptive, relaxed times—although such experiences can also be enjoyable, if we have worked hard to attain them. The best moments usually occur when a person's body or mind is stretched to its limits in a voluntary effort to accomplish something difficult and worthwhile. Optimal experience is thus something that we make happen. . . . Such experiences are not necessarily pleasant at the time they occur. The swimmer's muscles might have ached during his most memorable

race, his lungs might have felt like exploding, and he might have been dizzy with fatigue—yet these could have been the best moments of his life. Getting control of life is never easy, and sometimes it can be definitely painful. But in the long run, optimal experiences add up to a sense of mastery—or perhaps better, a sense of participation in determining the content of life—that comes as close to what is usually meant by happiness as anything else we can conceivably imagine (p. 3).

Csikszentmihalyi found that, whenever improvement of the quality of life is the goal, understanding the state of flow points the way to success. Whether in education, business, the arts, or—you guessed it—designing exercise routines for your clients, understanding how humans gravitate toward the flow experience is paramount to the success of your training program.

Quickly then, let's look at the criteria for the optimal flow experience. Much of it you have probably already figured out. However, it is helpful to define clearly what works for people and why. Csikszentmihalyi succinctly states it this way :

The optimal state of inner experience is one in which there is order in consciousness. This happens when psychic energy—or attention—is invested in realistic goals, and when skills match the opportunities for action. The pursuit of a goal brings order in awareness because a person must concentrate attention on the task at hand and momentarily forget everything else. These periods of struggling to overcome challenges are what people find to be the most enjoyable times of their lives. A person who has achieved control over psychic energy and has invested it in consciously chosen goals cannot help but grow into a more complex being. By stretching skills, by reaching toward higher challenges, such a person becomes an increasingly extraordinary individual (p. 6).

What we do as trainers, athletes, and entrepreneurs incorporates some of the most basic positive pleasures, as well as some of the most challenging disciplines, that life has to offer. We get a kick out of watching our businesses (and bank accounts) grow. We are challenged to use our creative energies when developing flow states for our clients to enter when they exercise, and then take great pleasure in seeing them become healthier and happier individuals. We strive to experience our own personal type of flow when we are particularly engrossed in our own athletic pursuits. We challenge ourselves daily to stay positive, current, open, fit, and available to our clients as they work to get in better shape. Great personal trainers have the ability to establish a feeling of flow in even the most resistant of clients as they guide them through their exercise routines. They understand that everyone, including those who may choose to deny it, has the primordial instinct, or need, to feel some kind of flow state on a physical as well as psychological level, and they are skilled at creating an environment conducive to achieving it.

The way these trainers guide their clients to reaching optimal experiences is by challenging them effectively—not so much as to overburden them, and not so little as to bore them. This involves establishing a personal "set-point" with each client. A set-point is a place where the client feels comfortable and from which he or she can proceed. Once a set-point has been established, the trainer has the freedom to develop realistic goals and a systematic approach to reaching those goals based on the client's individual needs. As the client achieves higher and higher goals, the trainer raises his or her personal set-point proportionally higher. When a client's envelope of ability is pushed a little further each session, it becomes easier for him or her to overcome even more difficult physical challenges. This could be something as simple as increasing the number of repetitions they do every other week, or pushing them to run an extra half-mile periodically. This, in turn, leads the client to feel more and more comfortable in the healthy flow state of a regular exercise routine. They begin to develop not only a stronger constitution, but also a certain confidence that they can do just about anything they put their minds to.

The workout, consisting of their effort, your training program, and your motivation, becomes one of the most important flow-producing activities of your clients' lives. It is but one of the ways they start to experience their own personal success.

Can you see now why your job is so complex? In addition to having good communication skills, you must also be able to motivate, cajole, admonish, inspire, and ever-so-skillfully guide your clients to a healthier way of living—all while helping them to maintain the personal flow state they've developed through your program.

Here are seven key points to remember when working to bring out the best in your clients:

1 Establish each client's personal set-point and use it to formulate an exercise program that will challenge him or her, not too much and not too little. Inspire your clients, through the challenge of your program, to strive for even higher set-points, thus allowing them to enter into their own personal flow state.

2 Share with your clients examples, stories, or mental images of times when you (or people you know) have experienced a flow state, and entice them to form their own personal feelings of happiness and deep concentration as they exercise with you.

3 Subtly infuse the goal of having an "optimal experience" into their exercise programs, and encourage your clients to seek this feeling in other activities as well.

4 Pursue healthy optimal experiences yourself. The more you experience them, the more effectively you can communicate them to your clients.

5 One of the specifics to enjoying a state of flow is the fact that it often comes after voluntary hard work. Emphasize this point with your clients: nothing can replace the satisfaction that comes from accomplishing a cherished goal after a period of concerted effort.

6 Savor your clients' accomplishments with them as their partner in health, and acknowledge the hard work they do. If it were easy, it would not be nearly as satisfying. Help them find their own personal "order in consciousness."

7 Understand that only through "order in consciousness" do people ever truly feel that they are the authors of their own destiny. When we endeavor to instill this mindset within our clients, we are actually helping to satisfy a universal desire of all human beings: the need to believe that they have control somewhere in their otherwise crazy lives.

Finally, let's recap the lessons that can save you time and money and spare you frustration and disappointment.

Lesson One: *Put your clients' success before your own.*

Lesson Two: *Remember the Matthew Effect: Success breeds success.*

Lesson Three: *Cultivate pleasure and flow states.*

2 *Creativity: The Key to Control*

S cientists have found that people (as well as other primates and species) become agitated, angered, stressed, fearful, and sick when they feel their lives are out of control. In your work as a personal trainer, you have no doubt noticed that one of your main goals is to learn how to assist your clients in regaining a natural and healthy control over their bodies. Creativity is especially helpful when you strive to achieve this goal. Why? Because creative expression is especially enjoyable. People are naturally drawn to it. Being creative and being in control go hand in hand, because when someone is being truly creative, he or she often feels "in control." Before going deeper into how creativity works for us as personal trainers, let's first learn why it works.

In Csikszentmihalyi's research, he found that "designing or discovering something new" is one of the most favored activities for people. He proposed a thought experiment to help us understand why humans are programmed to seek new discoveries, cultivate creativity, and feel they have control over their lives.

The thought experiment: Imagine with me that you are building an organism or artificial life form. Imagine that this organism's environment

is unpredictable and complex. How would you design it?
Csikszentmihalyi writes:

> You want to build into this organism some mechanism that will prepare it
> to confront as many of the sudden dangers and to take advantage of as
> many of the opportunities that arise as possible. How do you go about
> doing this? Certainly you would want to design an organism that is basi-
> cally conservative, one that learns the best solutions from the past and
> keeps repeating them, trying to save energy, to be cautious and go with the
> tried-and-true patterns of behavior. But the best solution would also
> include a relay system in a few of the organisms that would give a positive
> reinforcement every time they discovered something new or came up with
> a novel idea or behavior, whether or not it was immediately useful. It is
> especially important to make sure that the organism was not rewarded only
> for useful discoveries, otherwise it would be severely handicapped in meet-
> ing the future. For no earthly builder could anticipate the kind of situations
> the species of new organisms might encounter tomorrow, next year or the
> next decade. So the best program is one that makes the organism feel good
> whenever something new is discovered, regardless of its present usefulness.
> And this is what seems to have happened with our race through evolution.
> By random mutations, some individuals must have developed a nervous
> system in which the discovery of novelty stimulates the pleasure centers in
> the brain (p. 108).

In order for the whole group to survive, some individuals need to have a
heightened appreciation of creativity, as well as the more obvious drives
for food, procreation, and intimacy. The pleasure centers in most people's
nervous systems are programmed to be particularly stimulated when creativity, discovery, or exploration is part of their current activity. In short,
creativity is rewarding.

Let's look at how this relates to you as a personal trainer.

Both you and your clients have nervous systems that are stimulated by
the discovery of something new. In your clients, this manifests itself as the
need to discover new activities that will allow them to develop the healthiest, best-looking physique they can possibly have. What gets your nervous system excited is discovering the different ways of using exercise to
safely guide your clients into the bodies they've always wanted to live in
and helping them to cultivate different pleasurable experience associa-
tions as they do the work needed to get there. Once they associate exercise

with having a pleasurable experience, the next step is to creatively inspire them to break through their personal set-points and then establish new ones. Your ability to challenge them on a continual basis is what gives them the order in consciousness needed to enter their own personal flow state. Once you can get clients to experience not just exercise pleasure, which can be temporary, but exercise flow, which is lifelong, you'll be on the road to becoming the type of personal trainer that is in constant demand.

Many trainers fail because they don't understand this human need to be stimulated through creative challenges and new discoveries. After getting their clients to the point of feeling good about exercise, they may assume they've done their job. Interestingly, this is exactly the point where a lot of people drop out of their exercise programs because just feeling good quickly begins to feel boring. For clients to have any hope of sustaining the exercise habit for a lifetime, they need to be regularly stimulated through new challenges. This means establishing the momentum that comes primarily through consistent creative effort. Always remember that there is a very fine line between being comfortable and being bored.

You may be thinking: Is it reasonable to think that we can sustain this high a level of consistent creative effort in our clients and not burn them out? Is there any other weapon in our arsenal besides creativity that will enable to us to inspire our clients to keep exercising for the rest of their lives?

The answer to both questions is yes: you can keep your clients excited about exercising without burning them out, and, yes, there is another element that has the power to stimulate. Like creativity, it also has tremendous personal appeal because it is especially enjoyable. In your training business, it is something that you must learn to confront or you will end up compromising not only yourself but also the effectiveness of your program. On a personal level, it's probably something you've been dealing with for your entire life without realizing it. What is it?

The Force of Entropy

According to Csikszentmihalyi, the force of entropy is even more primitive, and, at times, even more powerful than creativity. He writes:

> This too is a survival mechanism built into our genes by evolution. It gives us pleasure when we are comfortable, when we relax, when we can get away with feeling good without expending energy. If we didn't have this

built-in regulator, we could easily kill ourselves by running ragged and then not having enough reserves of strength, body fat, or nervous energy to face the unexpected (p. 109).

This natural urge can and should (within reason) overtake each of us as needed. It regulates whatever it is that keeps us from frenetically overextending ourselves. It represents the down-time that allows us to park our minds in neutral and recharge our batteries.

Unless we are aware of how these two polar opposites of creativity and entropy fight for dominance in our day-to-day experience, we might fall prey to allowing entropy to rule the bulk of our activities. We are all balancing our activities between discovery or exertion and entropy or "taking it easy." Knowledge of this balancing act helps us understand how to motivate and support our clients as they vacillate between these two opposite needs.

Unsuccessful trainers tend to get bored with their clients, and with this business, because they allow themselves to become immune to the pleasures of discovering something new. They sink into mild depression after enjoying the pleasures of extended hours of entropy and actually become oversaturated with it. They get excessively comfortable in doing nothing, and this causes them to resent finally having to do something. They suffer personally, their businesses suffer, and the entire industry suffers because they lack the excitement to train people, even though training people is what they claim to do for a living.

Personal trainers who avoid excessive entropy (but also don't kill themselves with overextending their business pursuits or physical activities) are the leaders in this industry. They understand balance; they live balanced lives and they are able to teach an understanding of this concept to their clients.

In your work, you may have noticed something regarding creativity, entropy, and mild depression. When people are prompted simply to get out and do something, often any feelings of mild discomfort, sadness, or lethargy diminish or disappear altogether. They are replaced with the pleasure of discovering or doing something new or enjoying the thrill of getting to know new stuff. The unpredictable nature of discovery is very pleasurable indeed, and the savvy personal trainer takes advantage of the momentum established when his or her clients enjoy the pleasures of creating a new physique or future.

So this is the "macro" view: a quick overview of how our humanness has been designed and how it works. We will not choose to do anything unless it potentially brings us pleasure. Our work, our relations with clients, loved ones, and neighbors, our leisure, our generosity, our educational pursuits, all of these things have, to some degree, an element of pleasure associated with them. Otherwise, we would quickly lose interest or find ourselves bogged down with responsibilities as we trudge through the daily grind of being alive. We are motivated by pleasure!

Csikszentmihalyi has helped me understand this "pleasure principle" a little better.

Remember, you will be more successful in your business if you consistently share the pleasure of discovery with your clients. By cultivating this healthy outlook, you will be fortified in your efforts to assist them in avoiding destructive pleasures. As a guide to transformation, you will be visualizing the success of your clients and sharing your view with them as they progress. Soon, you will both have tangible proof of this grand and powerful view. Understanding how pleasure motivates us, how creativity and entropy fit in with other more obvious basic human drives, and how we can infuse this understanding into our business are all keys to our success as personal trainers.

Always remember that the real pleasure you'll get from this business will not, and should not, come from the money you receive, although I personally believe that there is nothing wrong with getting paid well for what you do. Your true wealth as a personal trainer will come from a natural, healthy sense of yourself, as well as the capacity to enjoy, get along with, and bring out the best in others. And—if I may be so bold—it will come from the ability to be happy with what you have created and accomplished.

Let's summarize how you can harness the power of creativity for your, and your clients', success:

🏃 *Know that as a personal trainer, your primary goal is to assist your clients in regaining a natural and healthy control over their bodies.*

- ☆ Understand the important role that creativity plays in the achievement of this goal.

- ☆ Implement creativity, not only when designing exercise programs but also in their application.

- ☆ Realize that "designing or discovering something new" is one of people's favorite activities. Use this fact to your advantage.

- ☆ Learn to balance your clients' need to be stimulated through creative challenges with their need to experience a certain level of "down time" or entropy, to rest and recover from their workouts.

- ☆ Remember that you must first be living this balance in your personal life for it to have any impact on your clients. Set a good example for them.

- ☆ Strive to make exercise a pleasurable experience for your clients by using discovery and creativity as well as entropy or relaxation.

3 *Understanding Your Market*

*W*ho your clients are, how they live their lives, what motivates them, what they look for in a trainer, and how they think about the process of exercising are all things you must consider when growing your business. This chapter will give you some thoughts and strategies about personal training as a business. Let's begin by taking a look at this ever-expanding market and how to tap it.

Before we can think of marketing our services to people, we must first identify who they are. A simple visit to the Chamber of Commerce in any city or town will yield a wealth of information about the people who live there. Chamber folks love the fact that you want to do business in their town and are more than happy to divulge the average income level, age, marital status, and recreational habits of the people who live there. With that information in hand, the next step is to contact any health clubs or recreation centers in the area and find out how many members each one has and how many of those members take advantage of personal training. By asking the right questions, you'll quickly get a realistic estimate of how many people in your area may be interested in and can afford a trainer.

Ninety percent of the clients you will train belong to a predictable socioeconomic class. Obviously, there will be exceptions to the rule, and the demographics of where you choose to establish your business, as well as the attitude of the community, will have a great impact on what type of clients you'll have. In certain parts of Florida or Arizona, for instance, the average client may tend to be over sixty and affluent. In Dallas or Santa Cruz, they may be younger and more working class. In Boulder, where I have my business, running, biking, skiing, hiking, and climbing are popular methods of relaxation. In some other parts of the country, the only reason people run is if they're being chased.

On the average, the typical clients who will need your services:

⚇ *are between 35 and 65 years of age;*

⚇ *have a steady income of over $30,000 a year;*

⚇ *can make the time to do some form of exercise, but may lack the self-motivation to work out consistently or at all;*

⚇ *have experienced a recent life change that caused them to reevaluate their body image and lifestyle;*

⚇ *are in a rut with their old exercise routine and need a new perspective.*

Once you target specific prospects within your area with the intention of selling them something, they become a Real Market. Advertising is nothing more than a method used for targeting prospects within your Real Market. The best advertising in the fitness industry is word of mouth. Please bear that in mind with each new prospect.

A Real Market can be whatever you want it to be. Perhaps you're going for one that is extremely defined, like all the former tri-athletes who participated in the 1987 Ironman and currently live in Whitefish, Montana. Or, you could go for a broader view, like all the overweight people over forty living in America. The clearer the picture of who your market is, the better you'll be able to create training programs tailored to their specific needs. Again, the ability to read and understand your market is where it all begins.

Know the Difference to Make a Difference

How do you turn a Real Market, just willing to entertain the thought of having you as their personal trainer, into a consistent weekly clientele? The answer starts with your understanding the difference between prospects, customers, and clients. A prospect is a person in a market who you believe would consider buying your service. When a prospect gives you money in exchange for one or two training sessions, he or she becomes a customer. A client is nothing more than a customer who has developed a mutually beneficial relationship with you over a longer period of time.

The truth is, a large percentage of the population simply doesn't have the time, knowledge, or motivation to exercise effectively on a regular basis, despite the fact that they're bombarded daily by studies and reports that say their lives may depend on it. Even after being taught proper form, technique, and exercise sequence, when left alone they either won't do it or will do it only halfway, with little enthusiasm and sloppy form. They tend to get frustrated, injured, and bored with exercise because they can't maintain the spirit that's required to make it work. For the average trainer, these are the people who'll make up the bulk of your clientele.

Given that clients are the indispensable elements of your business, you may ask where customers fit into the picture. The reasons I train customers, no matter how busy I get with my clientele, are: (1) some of my best client referrals have come from one- or two-time customers; and (2) I've had a lot of customers who initially just wanted to buy one or two sessions turn into clients.

Some customers may only need a little guidance and direction but can otherwise handle exercising on their own. These self-motivators may only need to check in every month or two for help in fine-tuning and updating their program, or you may see them just a few times to offer tips in getting their program started and never see them again. I'm not sure why, but self-motivating customers that I see on an occasional basis are responsible for well over half of all the referrals I get. Maybe it's because they already know the pleasures of fitness and are eager to share the experience. Always think of customers as an excellent source of word-of-mouth advertising.

Now that we can see the difference between a prospect or customer and a client, the next logical step is understanding how to turn one into the other. Obviously, you need to convince your prospects and customers that having you as their personal trainer will eliminate some of their problems, but how do you go about doing that? How do you develop the kind of trust it takes to become their long-term partner in health?

Straight from Your Heart to Their Heart

This may sound obvious, but you start by finding out everything you can about them before the first training session. The things you need to know are their expectations, needs, goals, fears, and failures. What do they want from you, and how hard are they willing to work at getting it? In the next chapter, I'll discuss in detail how to ask the right questions and get the right answers, but for now, I'd like you to just take a minute and think about what it would be like to see the world through the eyes of a certain type of customer.

This person is out of shape, unmotivated, and unhappy with his or her life. The best way to gain the level of understanding you'll need to help these customers is to picture yourself standing in their shoes, so do a little role reversal as you talk to them. Imagine what it would feel like to be in terrible shape, frustrated and powerless because every diet or exercise routine you've ever tried has failed. What would it be like to turn forty-five and come to the realization that you've never stuck with any kind of fitness program or consistent sport-like activity for more than a month in your whole life? What would it be like to feel hopeless and defeated in relation to your body?

To help these customers find ways to feel good about themselves and their bodies, you need a personal sense of their fears and frustrations, along with knowing what strengths they may possess and what motivates them. Role-reversing, along with empathy and the right questions, will enable you to quickly discover what will allow them to come out of a bad, resistant, helpless feeling and go into a motivated, vital, forward-moving feeling. Once you understand their problems, you'll be in a position to start charting their journey and inspiring them to take action. What follows are the tools you'll need to help build this empathy with every single person you train. If you use these tools, the market will be yours.

1 Motivation

What truly motivates a person to change? Standing over someone with a whip in one hand and a bullhorn in the other is certainly an effective means, but it usually lasts only as long as you can keep a person cornered in a room. How do you inspire that level of excitement even when they're not in your presence? What is the one thing that consistently motivates people to stay pointed in the direction of better health for a lifetime?

The answer is a belief in the future. This motivator is the underlying component of any movement towards growth and change. You must plant hope in the minds of your clients at the very beginning of your training relationship and cultivate it every time you see them. They must be convinced that their past does not equal their future. Clients not only need to let go of what hasn't worked up until then, but they must truly believe that they are very much in control of what lies ahead. This understanding must be in place for there to be any consistent movement forward.

To instill this belief in the people you train, you must first and foremost discover what brings them to you. Make a mental list of what they tell you in your initial consultation, and use this information to figure out what they need to feel about themselves in order to feel capable of moving into that very future you're both anticipating. Once a client believes that his or her body can look and feel better today than it did yesterday, and maybe even better tomorrow, he or she will naturally start to think in terms of realistic potential. Part of your job is getting them to let go of their past body image and start believing in a present and future body vision, as quickly as possible. Only then can you settle into your role as navigator of the boat instead of the person who just paddles it. To be a navigator in this industry, you must have the ability to motivate your clients with the feeling of confidence that what you offer is indeed a competent, effective, safe, and fun system of change. If they trust your approach and your support, they will feel motivated because they have the help they need, they have a future, and they have you, whom they trust, to guide them.

2 Anticipation: See Them Fit and Healthy

One of the most important skills you can develop is your ability to visualize the success of your clients even before they begin the process of reaching their goals. I always envision the person I'm training as a conqueror, a mighty person moving forward, always getting stronger and healthier. I see them conquering their feelings of weakness, apathy, uncertainty, and insecurity. I anticipate what they will look and feel like in the future, which allows me to create for myself a fresh mental image of who they wish to become. When I look at them, I actually see them exuding a super-positive attitude in their new strong body. I hold that vision for them. By always visualizing their new image, I'm also able to anticipate any needs that may arise as they progress and move closer to it. Thus, I'm always pointing them in the direction of more positive results.

Let me offer an example. People who may initially just want to lose weight are often afraid of building muscle because they don't want to get any bigger. Inevitably the ones with the least amount of muscle and the most fat will say something like, "Now Ed, I don't want to get all muscle-bound like those people in the magazines. I just want to trim down some and look good." They may not know that muscles burn fat when they are used in aerobic activity and resistance training, and they continue to burn it afterwards, even when you're sleeping. After a few months of training, when increased definition is noticed in addition to fat loss and heightened self-confidence, the same clients will most likely show interest in building even more muscle to gain more definition. Their vision of themselves will begin to change, and so will their attitude. This is an inevitable part of the transition people experience when going from fat to firm. To an intuitive trainer, this natural progression would be anticipated. To the client, it may come as a total surprise to realize they can actually increase their muscle size and definition but still look thinner.

As a trainer, you must also anticipate that your clients will become discouraged and feel defeated. See it coming. Read their bodies and faces, and ask questions. Be ready with the perspective that is true, the perspective of process, and be able to communicate and offer encouragement with genuine insight. Talk about your own experience or what you have witnessed in working with other clients.

Even your most enthusiastic clients will go through short periods of time when they just don't feel like exercising due to any number of different frustrations they could be experiencing in their lives. It's during these flat times that you as a trainer will experience the most challenging aspects of the job, because no one makes us work harder than the client who's having a couple of low-spirit days. This is the best time to talk about how far he or she has come in his or her journey and where the process is leading. Reestablish the client's original goal and commitment to reaching it, then describe the new image you see for him or her now, as well as in the future. This may have to be done on a regular basis. Remind clients that quite often the greatest progress springs from periods of feeling defeated.

People consider having a personal trainer because they are generally dissatisfied with some aspect of their lives. Perhaps they feel unattractive, unhealthy, or weak. Perhaps they have a strength goal they need help in achieving. Some people may come to training because they are obsessive about their appearance and perfectionists about looking a certain way. No matter what the scenario, your job as a trainer is always to point them in the direction of health and to show them how it is possible to feel good about themselves **as they get** stronger, rather than only **when they are** stronger. Health is a process, no matter how you look at it or how you approach it. Health is also a state of being and feeling that begins with your clients first accepting where they are, and then anticipating where they'll be headed in the future. As a trainer, you'll want to encourage that condition of vital, present-moment acceptance by offering your clients support at every leg of the journey.

3 Familiarization

The best way to support your clients is to get to know them as people, and the best way to do this is to familiarize yourself with how they live their lives. Find out the names of their spouses and children, the kind of cars they drive, where they work, any special problems they may be going through, or anything that is an issue in their lives. This shows that you acknowledge them on levels other than just the physical. It amazes me how many personal trainers don't realize the importance of this principle. By caring enough to remember important things about your clients, you actually become part of their lives. Once you become a positive part of someone's life, he or she will have a tendency to tell his or her family, friends, and coworkers about you, and the rest is history.

4 Get Jazzed!

Obviously, for you to motivate people you have to believe in yourself and your techniques. This level of true self-confidence must always be in place, because no matter how good an actor you may be, you can't fool people into thinking that you believe in them if you don't believe in yourself. Think of this belief in yourself as a pile of wood waiting to be burned, and then think of excitement and self-confidence as the sparks that will ignite the wood into a blaze. The key to turning customers into clients is in creating a relationship with them, and that relationship requires both logic and emotion. The trainer has to be passionate about him- or herself and the system of exercise in order for the customer to become emotionally engaged with it too. The emotional aspects of the relationship have to be mutual and reciprocal. This level of engagement makes clients out of customers.

How can anyone generate this level of excitement about personal training, or anything else, for that matter? The answer is in your attitude, your state of mind, and a power that grows out of the absolute belief that your system of fitness training really and truly helps people look and feel better. Enthusiasm, coupled with experience and self-confidence, sends a powerful message to a potential client. It says that here is a person who knows and loves what he or she is doing, who listens to me, and is someone whom I like! How can his or her system be anything but beneficial for me? Your ability to motivate people is a direct reflection of how excited you are about what you do.

5 Knowledge

To be convincing, to generate complete confidence, and to be motivating, you must become more than just knowledgeable about your field. You need to become an expert! Begin to think of what you do as a unique specialty. Then, do your homework and be prepared to answer any questions that might come up in regard to your specialty. Stay current by reading everything you can about it. Network with other experts in the field. Follow up with phone calls. Use the library for reference material. Go to trade shows and seminars. Pull it all together, and then get so involved in creating and mastering your own system of exercise that you could **actually sell yourself on it!** No joke!

It is only when you are thoroughly knowledgeable, creative, and on fire with inspiration about your system of exercise that you can successfully persuade prospects and customers to become clients. This attitude, coupled with experience and respect for people, is what allows your credibility to develop. Be aware of the difference between selling a genuinely helpful service and coming off like a pushy salesperson trying to sell a time-share condo in Cabo. Appealing to a person's higher instincts by using logic, reason, knowledge, experience, and the ability to understand and genuinely care about them leads to success in this business.

6 *Rehearsal*

You can be thoroughly knowledgeable, thoroughly prepared, have the best-equipped studio in town, and exude all the passion of a French general on Bastille Day, and still not be a successful personal trainer. You may be asking, "What more could it possibly take?" In order to take the next step, you must cultivate personal one-on-one skills. The most revealing way to assess your skills is to practice with someone who is not a close friend. Videotape the session. Then do the same thing with someone who is a close friend. Watch the two tapes with a critical eye and have a fourth person critique them as well. What you'll probably see in the first tape is that you seem a little uptight or ill at ease, while in the second one you'll most likely be calm and self-assured with the appearance of genuinely having a good time.

To put myself at ease while talking to prospects, customers, or clients, I'll sometimes imagine I'm having the same conversation with my best friend Mark. Our talks usually involve trying to convince each other about some issue in a non-threatening, friendly way by using all the logic and reason we can come up with. A good example of this took place a couple of months ago while we were discussing the politics of the late sixties and how they impacted our generation. Somehow, it came down to whether or not we should forgive Nixon for being such a shady character. My thought was that we should forgive him because of all the great music and jokes he inspired, plus the fact that he loved his wife and kids, opened a dialogue with China, liked Elvis, and, for a brief moment in time, gave us a scapegoat for all our nation's problems. I also pointed out that most politicians are kind of sneaky, and at least Nixon kept his sense of humor even when the whole country seemed to hate his guts. (Remember the great poster of him flashing the peace sign in front of the helicopter?) Mark, being a few years older than I, brought up Watergate, the Viet Nam War, Kent State, and a few obscure facts about Nixon's personal hygiene that he'd heard during a lunch break at the Washington riots of 1968. We went back and forth like that for the better part of an evening and had the best time.

My point is that the comfortable frame of mind I experience during these verbal exchanges allows me to talk convincingly about what I know without feeling intimidation or anxiety. People are generally at their best when they are in the comfortable environment of a group of friends exchanging ideas. If you can place yourself in that mindset and incorporate it into what you're saying, you'll find that discussing your system of exercise will come as naturally as talking to your friends. The conversation will take on an easy air of exchanging thoughts rather than that of a sales pitch.

The benefits of practicing this direct, yet laid-back, way of speaking are numerous. Perhaps the most important one is that it puts people at ease and minimizes any feeling of intimidation. This, in turn, opens the door to real communication. Through this open door you should quickly gain an understanding of any problems, needs, and other things that could benefit from your service. Once these have been established, you're in position to offer some real solutions. By comfortably asking the right questions, you'll also discover why a client's previous efforts have failed.

7 Understanding People and Their Problems

Remember, people don't buy products or services; they buy solutions to their problems. Even after asking all the right questions, the first two training sessions with new customers are sometimes difficult because they may not open up right away. This forces us to guess what their needs may be. Since problems are nothing more than unfulfilled needs, it becomes clear that our job is, first, about understanding what the customer's needs are, and second, about having the resources to fulfill them. The sooner you can familiarize yourself with the issues that seem to inhibit a customer's forward movement, the sooner you'll be in a position to help him or her move into better health and become a regular client. Another reason that I stress understanding the customer's problems is that if you don't understand them, they can quickly develop into your problems, especially if this customer becomes your regular client.

Clients' problems become your problems when they are chronically late to their sessions, when they don't take the program seriously, or when they constantly whine. Clients' problems become your problems when they don't assume responsibility for their bodies, when they expect you to miraculously transform them with little or no effort on their behalf, when they have major self-esteem issues, feel victimized by the world, or continually blame others for what goes wrong in their lives. These types of issues will make you crazy and inhibit you from doing your job if you allow them to.

Remember, your role involves not only putting people on customized exercise programs, but also being available to guide them through whatever obstacles may arise out of the process. This means developing the ability to keep clients pointed in the direction of better health, despite the fact that they may believe their lives are hopelessly screwed up in every other sense. It is within this journey to better health that most people find the hope and strength it takes to conquer other challenging aspects of their lives. Although exercise has a tendency to bring out the best in an individual, it also may temporarily bring out the worst, and you must be ready to deal with the good as well as the not-so-good. Your ability to empathize and work with clients on all levels is as important as any of the principles discussed so far.

When clients have personal problems that overshadow their ability to do your program, chances are it's because some key need of theirs (or quite often more than one) is not being met. The need to survive (to have food, shelter, clothing, and to reproduce), to feel healthy, happy, comfortable, loved, respected by others, and accepted by peers, friends, and family, are the most important aspects of a person's life. If any one of these is diminished or unattended to for any length of time, problems are bound to ensue. Look first at these areas if you wish to offer support, but beware of getting so deeply involved as to confuse professional boundaries. This could lead to the loss of the client.

The levels of a person's happiness, contentment and, in most cases, overall health are usually in direct proportion to the sense they have of themselves. That sense of self is almost always defined by love, respect, acceptance, fulfillment, and accomplishment. Without a sense of self, life becomes meaningless, for truly, the foundation for every life worth living, first and foremost, is the understanding and fulfillment of one's self.

I once had a client named Marsha whose life had become a meaningless array of daily routines and constant sadness. She was a prime example of someone who, at fifty, had lost a sense of who she was due to the fact that her kids had grown, her boyfriend was insensitive, her job was boring, and she didn't seem to fit in anywhere. By her own admission, she felt unloved, disrespected, unaccepted, and unfulfilled. She desperately needed to do something for herself, but every time she tried, by buying herself something or going on vacation, she'd feel guilty. On the advice of her therapist, she was willing to try exercise as a means of getting out of her head and becoming more in touch with her body, but she had no clue as to where to start.

For people like Marsha, having a qualified, sensitive personal trainer who understands them can be the key to opening the door to transformation. In the beginning, by getting her body to change even slightly, I was able to see a radical difference in Marsha's attitude, as well as her breathing, posture, and focus. By the tenth week of training, she could be described as nothing less than a warrior goddess. She not only regained a sense of who she was, but actually redefined herself by taking up new interests and activities, like tennis and power walking with a group of fit women her age. Within a year, she had a new job, a great body, a new boyfriend, self-confidence, and daily happiness. Although she might have come to some of these changes without my exercise program, I believe that it started the ball rolling. She had been in therapy for two years, but that in and of itself was just not enough to create the body/mind balance she needed.

What customers look for when shopping for a personal trainer is one who can help them define and fulfill themselves by giving them the tools to overcome certain physical limitations in their lives. What they end up paying you for is your ability to help them move beyond the frustration and disassociation that these limitations create. When people feel they look their best, when they actually know they're getting healthy, when they respect themselves and value their own efforts, when they finally move beyond previous limitations, then you have happy people, and satisfied clients who see you and your program as one of the reasons for their successful life. They will naturally want to achieve higher levels of health and happiness, and you represent a very important part of that evolution. You offer the solution to some of their biggest problems.

With the exception of physical rehabilitation, the most common reasons people give for starting an exercise routine are to lose weight; gain more strength, muscle mass, definition, and endurance; or to get better at a sport. What they're really saying is, "I want to look good and feel better about myself, but I don't know how to do it on my own." Success begins when you're able to convince them that your system of exercise is the answer.

8 Learning to Be a Successful Guide

Winning customers over involves convincing them not only that your system of exercise will meet their specific needs, but also that you have the ability to guide them safely to the results they desire. Being a guide involves making their journey as rewarding and individually challenging as possible by using their own strengths and weaknesses to determine how quickly or slowly they'll be negotiating the terrain. They must believe that you have a clear plan of action designed specifically to help them reach their goals, and that you've had experience helping others reach similar goals. A clear plan of action includes your ability to describe what the terrain looks like at the beginning, middle, and end of the journey you'll be taking them on.

The way you would hike with an eighty-year-old person would not be the same way you would hike with an eighteen-year-old, even if you took them both on the same trail. Although the trail would be the same, almost everything else about the experience would be different, including the pace, conversation, and reason for finishing. In order to make it interesting and challenging for you both, you'd have to consider their special needs, energy level, and reason for wanting to hike with you in the first place. The more people you train, or should I say, the more times you hike the trail, the easier it becomes to convince customers that you are the guide they need to have lead them.

9 Your Presentation

By the time you've tried to persuade ten people to buy your service, you will know more about presenting your system of training than any seminar could teach. Think about it. How could you possibly sell anything if you have no feeling for the market, no sense of current topics or phrases that get people excited?

When persuading people to become your clients, you must feel completely comfortable in your role and be able to put them at ease the minute you smile and shake their hand. Your presentation must be serious, yet light and informative without being too clever. That turns people off. Stress the benefits of your program, but don't fail to impress upon them that without a solid commitment from them, they will never reach their goal.

Your presentation must never be condescending or make people feel inferior because they may be out of shape. A lot of people may be intimidated by just being in a weight room or even being around you, so be gentle in your approach. When I talk to prospects, customers, or clients, I'm totally present. Direct eye contact indicates that my mind is focused only on them. As mentioned earlier, I also try to anticipate any fears or objections the person may have and directly address them as they come up.

Fears—of failure, of getting hurt, of not fitting in, of feeling foolish, and of being intimidated—are the major stumbling blocks that keep people from beginning a lifestyle of physical fitness and exercise. These fears are universal and know no boundaries. I've heard them expressed by teenagers as well as older folks, by men as well as women. In anticipating these fears and addressing them in your presentation, you're able to put them to rest before they become major issues.

10 Camaraderie: The Cure for Weight-Room Anxiety

If you choose to train your clients in a health club environment as opposed to a private studio, always introduce them to the regular exercisers that will inevitably be on similar schedules to theirs. Being familiar and comfortable with the surroundings means they're more likely to be long-term clients. Over a few sessions, they'll start to recognize the others who work out at the same time and develop a certain weight-room camaraderie. Your goal is to get your clients to feel like they're part of the gang of healthy people who work out every Tuesday morning.

Quite often, just having a personal trainer will eliminate much of the anxiety of starting a program. Working with a trainer provides a feeling of legitimacy and relieves the awkwardness of not knowing weight room etiquette. What most beginners need is a buffer between the reality of the weight room and their deep-rooted image of themselves. The most intimidating experience for out-of-shape people is to be caught in a room full of buff strangers in Lycra who seem to know exactly what to do. Even being alone in a weight room can make someone feel like a fool when he or she has no clue about what to do with the equipment or how to even start exercising.

11 How Not to Fail: Emphasize Quality, Quantity, and Specialty

By providing high quality and sufficient quantity in a unique, specialized service, you **absolutely will not fail** as a personal trainer, or anything else, for that matter! Higher quality means better service, more value, and a real awareness of what is being offered elsewhere. Know what your competition is doing so you can offer your clients something even better. In order to find out what my competition offered, I sought out one of the best trainers in my community and bought a few sessions from him. By having him treat me as though I were an inquisitive client, I was not only able to understand a client's experience, but, by picking his brain, I was also able to acquire three times as many exercises as I previously had in my repertoire. These two things were enormously helpful in developing my own system.

In seeking the counsel of a busy, successful trainer, as opposed to an overqualified, but not-so-busy one, I was able to discover workable tools I could apply directly to my service. Don't ask a loser for advice on how to be a winner. Most winners are happy to share their secrets of success with you, especially if you pay them. It's like saying, "I acknowledge and respect your success and I'd like to be just like you when I grow up." If this is done respectfully, the master won't feel threatened that the student is trying to compete with him or her directly.

Offering your clients sufficient or greater quantity means providing a full and complete training session that will leave them with the feeling that they've received more than their money's worth. At least in the early development of your business, always give clients more than your competition offers, at slightly less than your competition charges. Remember, you must first be worth more than you are paid if you ever wish to be paid more than you're worth. You can always raise your prices in the future, when you're so busy even your mother can't get hold of you.

A unique, specialized service is often one that is scarce or in limited supply. Obviously, there is an abundance of "qualified" personal trainers in this country, and yet true "quality" of service seems to still be in somewhat short supply. Although many qualified trainers do provide adequate service, a lot of them still can't seem to make a decent living and drop out of the business within a year or two. In reality, as the demand for our service increases, the chasm between adequate or mediocre trainers and outstanding and successful trainers will widen proportionately. At present, you can still make a few bucks even if you aren't excited or are bored with training people, as long as you're certified. This is because the public is still relatively naive about quality training versus mediocre training. In the future, however, as our industry moves from adolescence to adulthood, this will not be the case. The public, through experience, education, and a quest for superior service, will become increasingly selective in whom it chooses for personal training. The cream will naturally rise to the top, and those of us who are on top will not have gotten there by giving the public merely adequate or mediocre service. It will take a unique and specialized system of exercise that includes considerable variety, a plan of action, scientific background, excitement, creativity, communication, and results. By offering this type of service, you will be allowing the law of supply and demand to work for you.

Think of this as the outline for your success, or better yet, the foundation of your house of fitness. Here are the twelve essential building blocks of this foundation:

- *Understand the difference between a prospect, a customer, and a client.*

- *Know who your Real Market is. Tune into the demographics of where you choose to do business.*

- *Get to know each prospect by asking the right questions in the initial consultation. Do some role reversal and put yourself in their shoes.*

- *Use the answers they give you to visualize their future. Motivate them to share your vision.*

- *Get jazzed!*

- *Have the knowledge to back up your enthusiasm.*

- *Add confidence to your knowledge and enthusiasm by rehearsing your presentation with people you know, and people you don't know.*

- *Know that you represent a solution to some of your client's biggest problems.*

- *Understand that most problems people experience come from unmet needs. Establish and address these needs up front.*

- *Know how to tailor an exercise program to suit the specific individual needs of your clients. This clear plan of action makes them feel special and gives them confidence.*

- *Make a comfortable environment for your clients, wherever you train them. When training at a health club, introduce your clients to the "regulars" and allow camaraderie to develop.*

- *Know your competition. Save up your pennies and buy a couple of training sessions from the best trainer in town. Pick his or her brains and then add your own magic to what you already know works.*

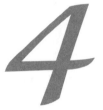

Personalities, Attitudes, and Body Types

Your ability to classify prospective clients will greatly enhance your power to quickly assess their needs. The reason for the classification is obvious: It saves us time. We simply do not have the luxury of spending hours second-guessing the real needs of a potential client, and we can't always count on them to tell us, or perhaps even to know. In the case of dislocated shoulders or broken bones, your direction is obvious, but what I'm talking about here are the kinds of needs that aren't so obvious—the needs that are unique to, say, men in their fifties with high blood pressure, or women who have just had babies. By categorizing prospects, I mean knowing that within certain groups of people lie similar needs or problems. Since different groups have different problems, as I've mentioned earlier, it behooves you to have lots of different solutions.

This is not about just putting prospects into boxes to make our job easier, but rather, using a wonderful tool for quickly understanding what motivated them to seek our help. Understanding this motivation is the key to knowing what options are open to us and how we are going to proceed. By knowing the traits that generally define a group, you'll be in a better position to address the needs of its individuals. The sooner we can get to the heart of people's problems, the sooner we can become a part of the solution.

The ability to categorize prospects correctly in your initial consultation is the first step to developing their exercise programs. Proficiency in this area has as much to do with your success as scientific background, creativity, enthusiasm, or any other principle discussed thus far. As always, experience is your best teacher.

For the sake of simplicity, I'll offer examples of some basic categories I might use when trying to establish why a potential client was compelled to see me. Let's start with the most important category—**attitude**—followed by the prospect's **gender, age,** and then **level of ability** (including any limitations). The reason this first category is the most important is that the level of a client's will is a direct reflection of how he or she feels about the work he or she is about to do, and it is through that feeling or attitude that he or she will either experience success or not.

A few words about attitudes: People perceive the experience of exercise on many different levels. I'm convinced that it's not in everyone's makeup to embrace exercise with the level of passion we trainers would always love to see. As a matter of fact, some people, no matter how hard they try, just plain **hate** to exercise. You can try a million ways to make it more fun, but if they don't have the spirit of excitement, the willingness to try to make it a good time, then exercise can potentially become just another nasty twice-a-week obligation. How do we work with folks in this category, who know they need to exercise and are willing to pay you for guidance, but can't stand actually going through the process? Obviously, all of us would love to have clienteles full of smiling, happy people who embrace exercise with the kind of excitement seen on Richard Simmons videos, but that's just not reality.

A good example of someone I've worked with in this category is my client Anne. After training Anne for about four years, I've come to know her as one of the most wonderful, caring, loyal, and lovable individuals I'd ever hope to meet. Her general outlook on life is upbeat and her overall demeanor is so accommodating and positive that she's truly a joy to be around. Her only problem is that she absolutely **hates** to exercise. You'd think that after training twice a week for four years she'd at least learn to like some aspect of it, but she doesn't. She mentally associates exercise with extreme pain and frustration, followed by brief moments of good feelings that usually come at the end of every session. To Anne, working out is right up there with going to the dentist.

When working with clients like Anne, I find it helpful not to lose sight of my established intent and always to stay focused on her goals and my responsibility to help her reach them. Please understand the distinction between intent and responsibility. As a professional trainer, my biggest responsibility is safely training her body to become more fit using the system of exercise I deem to be most appropriate. My intention is to make the journey as exciting and fun as possible, even if she doesn't want to get excited or have fun. Although I don't always see the fruits of my intention, I can't ever lose sight of or compromise my responsibility.

The best approach to use when working with clients who hate exercise is the same one you use when working with people who love exercise, and that is to think like a tour guide. Try to picture yourself as one of the rangers who guide tours through Yellowstone. For the most part, the tourists you deal with are friendly, happy folks who love having you tell them all the neat things about the park as you take them on the different nature hikes they've signed up for. Every once in a while, you'll run across the guy who only went on the hike because his wife dragged him along and who can't wait to get back to the Yellowstone Lodge to watch the baseball game on cable. Even though you may experience resistance in his attitude, the opportunity is still there to help transform him into a nature lover, or at least show him a different way of looking at the outdoors. Your job is about getting him through the hike as safely and happily as possible, knowing that, even if he doesn't emerge with flowers in his hair, he'll still be better off for having followed you through such a beautiful place.

By becoming the guide in your clients' journey to better health and by having the patience to really stick with them even when they dislike or are uncomfortable with the process, you'll find that you will experience your own type of transformation. You'll go from being a teacher of exercise to a motivating partner in growth. Above all, you'll want to leave space for this person to change by not judging or jumping to conclusions about how you think he or she should be.

By understanding the following additional categories and how to work within each one, you'll gain a more practical approach to guiding your clients to their desired results.

First, break each **gender** into these **age groups:** under twenty, twenty to thirty-four, thirty-five to forty-nine, fifty to sixty-five, and over sixty-five. Then, consider these three **levels of ability:** people in great shape who exercise on a regular basis; people in moderate shape who exercise sometimes but not consistently; and people in terrible shape who wouldn't know an exercise from an artery. Self-discipline can vary greatly from person to person, regardless of age or ability level.

The majority of prospective clients in your market will fall into one slot of each of the four categories, ending up with four traits for each person. You could encounter a fifty-six-year-old man in great shape with a good attitude, or a twenty-three-year-old woman in moderate shape with a bad attitude. Your logic, reason, and general approach would be different when discussing your program with these two individuals. Barring that rare person going through a sex-change operation who won't tell you how old he or she is, you should have no problem classifying most people who come to you for training. (This actually happened to a trainer friend of mine!)

The Fifteen-Minute Rule

Once you've classified a prospect, it becomes easier to connect with, make a plan for, and convince them that your system of fitness is their best bet. Sounds reasonable, right? The tricky part is getting all four things accomplished within the first fifteen minutes of your initial conversation.

This is what I refer to as the Fifteen-Minute Rule.

Most potential clients will simply lose interest if you haven't impressed them on several levels in this short amount of time. This initial talk we give not only enables us to establish our level of competence, but also gives the prospect confidence in knowing that we've heard them and have a clear plan of action. Blood pressure, fat caliber, VO_2 max, and heart rate testing should all be done after you've had your fifteen minutes of glory. At that point the prospect has already decided whether he or she is going to hire you or not.

The fifteen-minute rule works like this:

1 The first five minutes are spent classifying the prospect by the categories I just outlined: attitude, age, gender, and level of fitness.

2 The next five minutes are spent learning what his or her needs are and coming up with a few different program options to fit those needs.

3 The last five minutes are spent describing your plan of action and outlining just how your system of exercise is going to help the prospect reach his or her goal.

With experience, you'll develop an intuitive sixth sense that will allow you to know what the prospect wants and needs. Because some people do not communicate well or may not have a clear idea of what they need, you are at an advantage. Nothing impresses a potential client more than your ability to tune into his or her thoughts and articulate them with a clear and concise plan of action. With practice, you'll eventually be able to identify a person's needs just by watching how they walk, talk, and hold themselves.

People in search of quality trainers are looking for certain dynamics that include direct communication skills, confidence, applicable knowledge, and intuitive sense. Combine these four attributes with the fifteen-minute rule and you'll soon be hearing those fifteen words all good trainers love to hear: "So, when can you fit me into your schedule? I want you to train me."

Learn to Paint Pictures with Words

Successful trainers develop the ability to paint clear visual images for prospects by using the terms and phrases of our profession. When used properly, these words enhance a trainer's ability to understand the needs of potential clients. Visual images created through word association enable us to cut through the small talk and get down to what the prospect really expects from us.

Some examples of these phrases are: more definition, weight loss, increased endurance, less fatigue, more strength, lower heart rate, more efficient metabolism, lower stress level, increased immunity, increased mental clarity, better overall health, stamina, tone, cut, lean muscle mass, and better attitude. Of course, these phrases are nothing less than the benefits of being fit. When included in your initial conversation with a prospective client, these words help to create a physical image the person can visually grasp. When you hit on one they like, their eyes will light up and they'll say something like: "Yeah, I want that, too!" (Of course a quality trainer would never promise something he or she couldn't deliver.) Nevertheless, by being aware of prospects' reactions to your words, you'll be able to make a note of what things are most important to them and quickly address and incorporate them into your plan of action. When the time comes to actually sell your system in that last five minutes, you'll have the edge.

This technique is very efficient because you waste no time trying to sell prospects things they don't find important. Instead, the time is spent customizing a program that fits them like a glove, based on the information you've gathered by watching their reaction to the picture you've painted. It also allows you to address any questions they may have concerning metabolism, stress, or weight loss. I know this is a lot to cram into fifteen minutes, but with a little practice it becomes second nature and you'll begin to know instinctively what questions to ask, and how to ask them. For example, people over fifty may respond better to terms like less fatigue, lower blood pressure, lower heart rate, and better overall health, whereas folks between twenty and thirty-five are more likely to be looking for more definition, lower stress level, more strength, increased endurance, and/or weight loss. A thin person is not going to be concerned about losing weight, and a heavy person is obviously not going to want to gain more, although both may want more definition, strength, or stamina. People in great shape may feel as if they're being patronized if the words you use imply that they're totally ignorant of how the human body works, whereas people in less than great shape may need you to explain the most fundamental exercise concepts to them. You may have to give them a course in Beginning Fitness 101.

Everyone who walks through your door will have specific, individual needs that may take a little work to uncover, as well as general, obvious needs that become apparent simply by analyzing their body type. An important aspect of your evaluation is trying to understand how the client feels about his or her body now and how he or she would like it to look and feel in the future. People over sixty routinely do not want to look like Arnold, whereas people under thirty may want you to point them in that direction. In order to be supportive of people's different needs, you must be alert and conscious of the individual at all times. Do not make assumptions without first reading your prospect and carefully listening to the messages he or she is sending, both verbal and non-verbal.

This concept of listening for a niche or void and filling it with your unique service is the cornerstone of any sale, whether you're selling fitness, knowledge, snowcones, or tennis shoes. Although this seems obvious, I am always amazed to see how many personal trainers fail to recognize these basic rules of marketing.

Keep Them Interested

Common errors when dealing with prospects include not listening to them, as well as selling them "cookie cutter" exercise routines when they really need customized programs. A "cookie cutter" routine uses the same series of exercises for everyone with little regard for body type, age, or ability. Not much thought goes into these routines and often the only things that vary are the repetitions and weight resistance. This paint-by-numbers way of training quickly becomes predictable and monotonous for the client and just plain boring for the trainer.

Customized programs, in contrast, include variety, excitement, and some thought on behalf of the trainer. The very nature of customized programs is that they are constantly changing and adapting to the client's body as it changes and adapts to its new way of feeling and looking. As your clients' bodies change, so will their needs, and that is where the job gets fun because you get to start being creative. Creative trainers are just like creative people in any profession. They do not become stuck in outmoded thinking. They are always present and vital. They are models of what the client wants to become. They're always trying new things and thinking up new ways to challenge their clients using the unlimited combination of exercises at their disposal. Great trainers are visionaries; weak trainers are "cookie cutters."

After a person becomes my client, I make a point of not letting them know from one session to the next what I'm going to have them do.

Although I can't help repeating certain exercises, particularly with clients who do more than two sessions a week, I always endeavor to make my training sessions as varied as my clientele.

Offering a variety of exercises that work the same muscle groups in different ways will keep your practice from getting stale because it enables you to continually select new options for your clients. Variety keeps you out of the very predictable "If it's Thursday it must be bench press" mentality, and gives you the unique advantage of being able to customize a new workout each and every time you see someone.

Think of how much more excited and motivated your clients will be if you surprise and challenge them each session. I know this goes against the conventional wisdom of writing down and charting every repetition of every set an individual has done and then letting them take these "progress charts" home like some form of little reward for being good. Experience has shown me that when clients are encouraged to keep a record of every repetition they do, there is a good chance they'll become addicted to keeping written records and using them to gauge their success. This is counterproductive in that it places too much emphasis on numbers and not enough on the person's actual physical changes. I've seen people get so caught up in keeping a record of past workouts that if they forgot to bring their progress chart to the gym they would simply turn around and go home, because they couldn't remember the sequence of their last workout and heaven forbid they should do anything spontaneously.

As a trainer, I always write down (in my personal note pad) everything I've had the client do in previous sessions. This not only allows me to vary their next session accordingly, but also helps keep things fresh and exciting, because I'm the only one who knows what the next session will involve. Taking this approach puts me in control of training logistics and allows the client to concentrate on more important things, such as tuning in to their body and noticing the changes that are taking place as they get increasingly fit. You will see a greater level of success in this business if you keep your clients focused on reaching their physical goals and seeing their bodies change, instead of seeing how many more reps they can do compared to last week.

Clients, especially those in moderate shape between the ages of thirty-five and fifty, have a tendency to identify more with the process of getting fit than the goal of being fit. Generally speaking, the better shape a client is in, the less need they have to identify with and compare progress charts. Fit people have fun when doing activities such as running, biking, or lifting weights. Unfit people don't have as much fun doing physical stuff, so they chart and compare everything they do, thinking it will add some magical element of fun to the activities they already don't like doing. It doesn't! When training new clients who have never exercised, I do allow them to keep a record of what we've done for the first few weeks if they really feel the need. It gives them something to look forward to until their bodies start to change, at which time I redirect their focus and place it on how they're looking and feeling. The sooner I can build their confidence, the easier it is to wean them off the need to compare charts and get them into feeling how differently their clothes are starting to fit.

This practice makes sense in other professions too. Roger, my mechanic, will inevitably explain to me what he's going to do before he fixes my car. He does not, however, allow me to be in on the process of fixing it by giving him advice, or even watching him work. Once I explain the problem, I trust him to do a great job and give me the results I need. Likewise, an airline pilot may tell you the route and altitude at which you'll fly, but does not invite you to take the controls of the plane. You care more about whether you've reached your destination safely and relatively on time.

Success: First Personal, Then Financial

I know I'm a success in my personal training business when clients tell me that they can't believe how much more strength they had in their tennis serve, or that they rode an extra five miles on their bike because of the cardio and leg work we've done. Or, in the case of elderly clients, I know I'm a success when I hear that they don't feel as much pain in their hips while walking, or when a middle-aged client who's had a weight problem his entire life can now see his shoes without bending over. This type of feedback is what makes personal training a rewarding profession. It is the means by which to gauge the real success of our business. Only when you've reached the point where people rave about the physical results they've seen through working with you will you start to see the kind of financial rewards that this profession can offer. Focus your attention on helping your clients move through life with as little physical impediment as possible in the healthiest body possible, and your monetary success will follow.

Before summarizing this chapter, I'd like to leave you with a two-thousand-year-old quote from a guy named Paul who, unknowingly, just happened to write the coolest advice for building a clientele. What he wrote was, "I have become all things to all people" (1 Corinthians 9:22). Being both Jewish and a Roman citizen enabled Paul to move comfortably between these two diverse cultures that were at odds with each other, and still stay alive long enough to get his message of love across. Granted, both groups did at times throw him in jail and beat the hell out of him, and the Romans did eventually kill him, but he was still able to accomplish his mission because he understood both cultures. His knowledge of language and customs, as well as his ability to talk comfortably to people on all different levels of society, enabled him to truly know and be accepted by all kinds of people. (Of course, a little help from upstairs didn't hurt.)

Obviously, you'll never be "all things to all people," but as a great personal trainer, your success will be in direct proportion to your knowledge, understanding, and acceptance of all the different types of people who come to you for training. Your reputation as a trainer who listens and cares about your clients will spread like wildfire, and you'll need a secretary to keep track of all the people who will want to train with you.

Summary

🏃 *Develop the ability to quickly read people and categorize them according to gender, age, level of ability, and attitude.*

🏃 *Master the Fifteen-Minute Rule.*

🏃 *Know what people look for when interviewing personal trainers: direct communication skills, total confidence, and applicable knowledge.*

🏃 *Know how to create a visual image for the prospect using the words of our profession. Notice how they respond to these phrases and incorporate them into your plan of action.*

🏃 *Don't promise results you can't deliver.*

🏃 *Learn to recognize, analyze, and discuss the client's less obvious needs as well as his or her obvious needs.*

🏃 *Incorporate into your system a variety of different exercises that work the same muscle groups in different ways. Customize a new workout each and every time your client comes in.*

🏃 *Don't let your clients become progress-chart junkies.*

🏃 *You take control of training logistics. (Keep a record of their training sessions in your personal note pad.)*

🏃 *Strive to be "all things to all people" in the fitness world. You'll be in great company.*

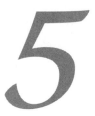

The Resources of Successful Personal Trainers

*The secret of success is to decide what you want out
of life and go about gathering together the means
and materials by which to achieve that end.*
—Aristotle

I love this quote because it succinctly describes two of the most important elements of successfully reaching any goal: deciding what you want, and then applying your resources to get it. Pretty straight-forward, huh?

Assuming this secret applies to everyone, including personal trainers, then logically, the next two questions should be: what are our resources, and how do we apply them to building successful training businesses?

As trainers, our three most valuable resources are:

🏃 *our mind/body balance,*

🏃 *our level of visibility, and*

🏃 *the people in our resource network.*

So many trainers fail to recognize these resources that they simply have to be discussed. What is most important is your ability to establish a balance between your own mind and body; in other words, your mind needs to be as sharp as your body is fit. You need, at least initially, a high level of visual exposure. In addition, you must surround yourself with a network of positive allies if you ever wish to succeed and be happy as a trainer.

Begin by picturing your training business as a steel-reinforced building, with your clear mind and healthy body as the solid ground upon which its foundation rests. Next, think of your allies as the structure's walls and roof, and its windows as your level of visibility. Eliminate any one of these elements, and your building will be compromised either structurally or esthetically.

Let's start by discussing the solid ground beneath your foundation.

Resource One: Your Mind and Body

In addition to all the obvious ways that a connection between a healthy body and a clear mind can assist you in your role as a trainer, perhaps the most important one is the example it sets for your clients. One reason people will choose to work with you, and not with other trainers, is that they feel you've reached a certain balance in your life that they find appealing. They may compliment you by saying they want their bodies to look like yours, but what they're really hoping to achieve is the feeling of comfort and satisfaction that you seem to exude in relation to your body—and your life. This mind/body balance, or connection, is manifested in your spirit, the way you communicate, your level of confidence, your attitude, your physical presence, and the overall feeling people experience being around you. It attracts clients to you because it taps into their primordial instinct to associate with the healthier, happier members of our species. If you're not healthy and happy, they're not going to want to be around you. Once they can see you have the feeling of health, both mentally and physically, your clients will want to know how you were able to develop it, and then they'll want you to teach them how to achieve it. These are the things that make you a valuable commodity to people who are searching for ways to increase their chances of having a better quality of life.

Successful trainers continually refine and embrace the feeling of healthy mind/body balance, and they work on these two areas inter-dependently. Mediocre trainers tend to spend more time making their bodies look good and focusing on their own sports, while spending disproportionately less time working on their minds, communication skills, and exercise system.

Begin to polish these areas of your professional life by learning to emulate people who have achieved incredible success and recognition in the fitness world. Study people like Jane Fonda, Arnold You-know-who, and Bob Greene, all of whom comfortably manifest confidence, grace, health, peace, and success whenever we see them. Although having their bodies wouldn't hurt, what is perhaps just as important is your ability to think and be like them. By reading their books, viewing their tapes, and studying how they developed their successful attitudes, you'll subconsciously begin to reach for your own higher levels of success.

Unbalanced Minds and Bodies: What Goes Wrong?

I'd like to talk a little about how an unbalanced mind and body perception can cause your clients problems, not only when they start your program, but also as they progress in it. I believe most of the negative issues that people have around exercise are directly rooted in a distorted view they have of themselves, as well as the subconscious belief that their minds and bodies are somehow separate. People with distorted images of themselves tend to live so much in their heads that they forget they even have bodies. Or else they're so obsessed with their bodies that they focus on them to the exclusion of other things. This compartmentalized mentality is the common denominator that links together most people who experience negative, frustrating results from exercise. You'll find it in people who are extremely apathetic towards exercise, even though they continue to do it, as well as in those fitness junkies who are addicted to exercise. People addicted to working out have such a need to see themselves as a different body type that they often exercise in lieu of having hobbies, social contacts, recreation, and happiness. What they are really addicted to is trying to change how they think their bodies look, as well as experiencing higher and higher levels of muscle-induced brain endorphins. Everything else in life becomes secondary. Many anorexic people fall into this category.

Another extreme example of how distorted self-images can wreak havoc on a person's life is the addiction to immediate personal sense gratification. People in this condition tend to methodically torture themselves through indulgence in drugs or alcohol, food bingeing and/or purging, living in a chronic state of either entropy or overexertion, and generally doing anything that will bring immediate pleasure, regardless of the long-term consequences. Through denial and justification, they create the detachment needed to feel comfortable and at least look good, outwardly, all the while living in their self-imposed, destructive little hells. Many people suffering from bulimia and/or anorexia nervosa fall into this category.

Although you may never directly experience either of these extreme scenarios in your practice, you should still be aware that they may be the root of much of the anxiety and frustration you will experience as you work with clients. Distorted self-images can affect all age groups and genders, and sometimes the results overlap with each other in the process. Some bulimics become fitness junkies and some anorexics become apathetic couch potatoes. Not only do both groups exercise for the wrong reasons, they're never quite satisfied with the results they get because they didn't have a realistic image of themselves, or the process, to begin with.

When you encounter these types of individuals, if you're not careful, you can find yourself spending a disproportionate amount of time trying to convince them that their bodies really don't look the way they think they look. Frustration can rule these training sessions, because the void these clients think they're filling with exercise isn't about health or fitness, but about an insatiable need to see their bodies differently. This type of void can't be filled, despite the fact that they may be able to run 40 miles and do 500 crunches a day. Nothing is more challenging than working with potential anorexics who only feel alive when they're running and starving, compulsive jocks who are unhappily addicted to resistance training, overweight people who exercise to justify their food bingeing, or former steroid users who wish to stay off drugs and still maintain the massive muscles they had when they were using them.

Over the years and through countless discussions with people about how they see themselves, I've come to appreciate how much of the fitness feeling really is a state of mind. The enormous part the mind plays in allowing a person either to enjoy life or to feel miserable can be seen in the smiling face of a fit-though-handicapped skier after finishing a Special Olympics race. It also shows itself in the tortured look of an ultra-distance runner with three percent body fat who jogs and does weights every day, but still never feels satisfied or healthy.

As trainers, the way we can be most effective when working with distorted-image clients is, at least in the beginning, to take the emphasis off how they see their bodies and encourage more of the feeling aspect of the work. This is why initiating the mentality of flow at the onset of your relationship is important. The reason is that flow is a feeling state, and clients need to feel different before they'll put in the time it takes to look different. Use your peaceful, clear mind and healthy body as an example of what it's like not to be in the middle of a mind/body struggle. Once they can experience what it's like to really feel healthy and balanced, a certain peace takes over and they'll start to look at exercise as more of a positive choice, rather than an addictive daily battle. As you guide clients through this transition, using yourself as an example, their bodies will naturally begin to change with minimal risk of injury or mental turmoil. In short, your goal is to get your clients feeling good about their exercise routines and keep them feeling good for the right reasons. You may very well be the only healthy guide or example they've ever worked with on this level, and this responsibility should not be taken lightly.

In working with clients who come in more than once a week, you will also notice that a certain exasperation can set in if you try to accommodate or overlook every one of their changing emotional needs and habits. These things can change literally from session to session, and you'll need to develop, within reason, the ability to adapt your program to them without straying too far from your day's agenda. If the client happens to be crisis-oriented and stressed when he or she comes in, you'd want to structure his or her workout in such a way as to calm him or her down. Your demeanor and approach would be completely different than, say, if he or she were to come in half-asleep and lethargic, in which case you'd obviously try to wake the client up and energize him or her. Again, you set the pace for the session by first staying grounded in your mind and body, then establishing what the client's physical and emotional needs are for that day. You may do the same exercises in either case, but the overall session would have a completely different feeling to it. In reality, this business is just as much about working with a person's mental fitness as it is about helping to increase his or her level of physical fitness.

Here is an example of how the varied and changing emotional states of my clientele could have made me insane a few years ago, had I not had the right perspective. My Tuesday morning schedule in 1995 went something like this: At 8:00, I'd train Anne, who hated to exercise and made me feel like a dentist pulling teeth. (I talked about her in Chapter 4.) At 9:00, I'd train Harry, an upbeat athlete who loved sports and loved training for them. Working with Harry was a pleasure, because he exercised for the right reasons and his attitude was always right on.

At 10:00, it was Tim, who also seemed to like the work and had a good attitude, but had the passive-aggressive habit of arriving twenty minutes late for his sessions. Cramming a full hour of exercise into forty minutes left me feeling exhausted and frustrated. I eventually had to fire him. Then, at 11:00, it was Susan, who liked lifting weights, was always on time, and had a great attitude, but never did the follow-up aerobic work that I needed her to do on the days she didn't work with me. In short, she had great muscles, but remained overweight and frustrated because, by itself, the resistance training we did wasn't enough to burn her fat. At 12:00, it was Rhonda, who I now realize was probably an exercise-compulsive anorexic. Training her involved carefully holding her back for fear she'd hurt herself, while trying to convince her that, at 97 pounds, she wasn't fat.

Each of these five clients required a complete change of mental state in order to give each one a safe and complete training session. Without my ability to stay grounded and adapt to their individual nuances without compromising the program, I'm convinced I would have lost it and quit.

You can't help clients develop healthy mindsets about exercising their bodies until you cut through their armor. Part of the way you do that is through positive encouragement, motivation, understanding, your own example, and your ability to adapt to their changing needs. You don't have to be a mind reader in order to help clients have a more positive image of themselves, but you do need to develop a sense of how their hearts and minds can change from day to day in order to create the balance it takes to start.

Exercise is perhaps the healthiest way a person can work through the daily challenges of life, but it only works if he or she is at least trying to establish a healthy mind/body balance. In the process of helping a person reach this balance, you'll inevitably come up against insecurity and vanity, which are both issues of the mind and yet directly affect the relationship a person has with his or her body. Successful trainers not only help people rise above their insecurities, but also help them channel their vanity into a more productive form of energy, such as emotional and physical self-confidence.

What is vanity anyway? The *Oxford American Dictionary* defines it as "conceit, especially about one's appearance." Vanity is interesting in that everyone has a little of it, including people who live totally unfit and sloppy lives. I've met people who are self-proclaimed couch potatoes with appalling diets, who have never exercised a day in their lives, and yet are actually vain and conceited about their unhealthy lifestyles and appearance!

Let's face it, we're in the business of helping people reach a higher quality of life through physical fitness, and that involves not only working directly with their bodies, but also with the images they have of their bodies. It's impossible to work with the sometimes deep-rooted images a person may have about his or her body without coming face to face with the many sides of vanity. Clothing manufacturers, car dealers, interior designers, hair stylists, photographers, the movie industry, and other aspects of culture actually set the outward appearance standard for vanity in the world. We personal trainers have the opportunity to help create an internal balance in peoples' lives by working with vanity on a healthy, more productive level. Instead of working from the outside in, we work from the inside out. In and of itself, the fact that a person can buy a new Mustang and live in an expensive house will not bring happiness. Throw in a peaceful mind, a healthy body, and a great relationship, and the whole equation changes.

A little vanity is not a bad thing if its basis is the external manifestation of an internal peace, health, and happiness. Any time a person commits to making positive changes in his or her life, vanity, in some form, is usually an influence in that decision.

Looking Inside Yourself

You must first assess every aspect of your own life before you can help others make positive change happen in their lives. This includes looking at your own vanity as well as your lifestyle, self-image, and normal frame of mind. To some extent, being vain is part of being human. Only when it's taken to the extreme does it stifle a person's growth and cause anxiety. When viewed from this perspective, vanity can be used as a tool or stepping-stone to more positive things such as good health, peace of mind, and a better self-image.

Being a successful trainer means having the ability to guide clients through vanity, to physical/mental self-confidence. It is your responsibility to make the transition as smooth as possible, and the best way to accomplish this is by offering your own clear mind and fit body as an example of what your clients can also achieve. The next step is to give them proper guidance to make their own healthy lifestyle changes. When people see that you have taken the time to bring your own body and mind to a healthy place, they will naturally gravitate to you, because you represent the hope that they, too, can reach their higher potential.

I find it interesting that clients can so convincingly express the desire to see these changes take place in their bodies, and at the same time be so resistant or even fearful of putting forth the effort it takes to make them actually happen. The fear of changing daily lifestyle routines can scare a lot of people into complacency, unless you can convince them that the changes you'll be taking them through are safe and will ultimately lead to happiness. By sharing past experiences of your own evolution and the changes that you may have gone through in getting fit, you'll make it easier for your clients to experience the changes they'll be seeing and should anticipate as they continue in your program. You need to be a shining example of what the human body and mind can achieve through hard work and the willingness to change, and you must be able to create a safe environment in which your clients can do the same. I believe that is where real success lies—yours as well as theirs.

> *I eat change for breakfast.*
> —Phil Knight, President of Nike

Resource Two: **Visual Exposure**

The next resource to consider is visibility. The two key elements of this principle are: contact with large groups of people, and your ability to be seen training individuals consistently.

To build a large clientele in a relatively short amount of time, you must be exposed to lots of people on a regular basis. By initially working at a busy health club that is popular and has a good reputation, as opposed to a smaller neighborhood club that may have a limited client base, your profit potential will grow by leaps and bounds. The job may be harder to get and may require more than one certification, but the exposure is worth the extra work. Although it may be easier to find jobs at the smaller clubs, you'll have a harder time building a clientele for yourself, unless you're taking over someone's clientele or there is one already in place. People who are in the market for personal trainers tend to gravitate toward bigger, more established health clubs due to the fact that they seem more legitimate. Once established, you can always move your clientele to a more comfortable, less crowded environment. If you've already gotten a job at a popular facility, the next step in the road to your success is to have people see you training clients!

"But I have no clients, Ed! How can I look busy training clients when I have no one to train?" Good question! The secret here is to **act** as though you have a clientele, even if you don't. I am not kidding. Bring in your friends, family, acquaintances, or even coworkers, and offer to train them for free. You'll not only hone your skills and keep yourself from getting bored, but others will start to notice the fact that you're busy and will want to seek your counsel. This accomplishes two things: it allows prospects to see you interacting with "clients," and it lets you work out the bugs in your system without ruining your reputation. The more active you appear, the more prospect response you'll get. One-third of my original clientele was established through word of mouth. Two-thirds of them were people who saw me training someone else at the recreation center where I worked, and after the session, approached me to talk about their needs.

People who frequent health facilities have a tendency to be a little on the voyeuristic side. Although no one ever admits it, everyone checks out everyone else's body and form of exercise, and then compares them to their own. To a trainer, this can be a great asset. The advantage to you is that every time you're training someone in a health club setting, there's a good chance other people are noticing how you interact, your level of knowledge, and generally how you conduct the session. They'll also notice any changes your clients' bodies go through as they continue to work with you. Having people see you in action, working your system with clients, is perhaps the best and cheapest advertising you can do. Think of this high level of exposure as the spark that ignites the fire that becomes word of mouth. I realized this principle several years ago when I began to notice that the more people witnessed me working with others—in any capacity—the more people inquired about training with me. I also noticed that those trainers who sat around looking bored and reading muscle magazines had a tendency to stay in that dormant state and never get any clients. The irony was that a lot of those trainers had more technical knowledge than I did. The only difference was that I was in motion, still hungry to learn, and they were stagnant, having already learned it all.

Resource Three: Your Network

Another wonderful resource for developing a great clientele is your ability to network. Any successful individual will testify to the importance of networking in the achievement of their success. What they may not tell you is how amazed they were to see the different sources, frequently unpredictable, by which it drew opportunities to them.

You must wake up every morning with the intention of treating every contact you make as though he were the President asking your opinion about how to trim down those thunder thighs of his. Whether you believed in his politics or not, you'd still show him the utmost respect and try to impress him, because of the obvious fact that if he liked you, you'd end up with more clients than you could shake a stick at. Remember: That little unassuming sixty-year-old woman who asks your advice on what to do about the pain in her hip just may turn out to have a son or daughter in the White House someday—or at least have that kind of an influence on your business. You just never know.

Case in point: Several years ago, I met a grumpy man in his sixties who was under doctor's orders to start exercising, but just plain hated the idea of having to do so. I got the feeling he didn't particularly like anyone, myself included, although that didn't stop him from frequently asking my advice about exercise and diet as they related to his condition. This guy was so crabby and seemingly ungrateful that, at times, I had to bite my tongue to stop myself from telling him what I thought of his attitude— not to mention the fact that I was giving him the advice for free. To make a long story short, I did not pursue this man as a training client. Patience is one thing, but this guy would have made my life miserable.

The lesson here is that, ironically, in his own cranky way he actually did like me and ended up persuading his son (who also didn't think his father liked him) to come and talk to me about getting himself on an exercise program. The son, Jim, had a great attitude and became one of my best clients over a two-year period. He ended up referring me to several other prospects, including his supervisor, Hank, who just happened to be a member of a group of senior male joggers who all had great leg muscles and skinny upper torsos. I became the upper-body resistance trainer for the group, specializing in their arm, chest, back, and shoulder muscles. Not only did Mr. Grumpy inadvertently refer me to perhaps ten new clients, he also taught me a valuable lesson in patience, control, and the power of networking. Looking back, I'd have to say it was a very positive association. He got some free advice and I got some new clients and a few great lessons.

Because of that experience, I decided not to take for granted anyone who wants to talk about fitness. I never miss the opportunity to enthusiastically discuss my profession with anyone who seems interested, because opportunity has a way of showing itself when you may least expect it. You just don't always know whom you're talking to.

Networking is more than just handing out your business card to everyone you encounter in the course of your day. It's even more than being ready, at the drop of a hat, to explain what you do and how you do it to anyone who shows interest. Networking has more to do with the power you create when you think a certain way (back to the mind/body connection). This power, when applied to your attitude, has a magical effect on your ability to draw positive things into your life. You'll know you're beginning to reach the frame of life I speak of when you notice an actual network of positive allies starting to surround you.

If cultivated, this group of allies will eventually become what Napoleon Hill described in his book, *Think and Grow Rich,* as a "Master Mind Alliance." This is a group of like-minded people with whom you meet on a regular basis for the purpose of sharing experience, education, and specialized knowledge. This alliance creates a positive charge that is mightier than the negative forces the individual members encounter during the regular course of their lives. It's a success support system that helps its members gain more confidence and strength through constant, sustained support and the exchange of ideas. Think of it as a practical method of applying the assets of others to whatever end you may wish to pursue through a mutually beneficial association. It is networking at its finest!

> *When two or more people coordinate in a spirit of harmony, and work toward a definite objective, they place themselves in position, through that alliance, to absorb power directly from the great universal storehouse of Infinite Intelligence. This is the greatest of all sources of power.*
>
> —Napoleon Hill

When enthusiastic minds are united in harmony with singleness of purpose, there is brought into being the most powerful influence known. What is created is what Hill refers to as the "Infinite Intelligence." This is what Henry Ford tapped into when he came up with the idea for the V-8 engine, where Walt Disney went when he got the inspiration to create Disneyland, and where Mary Kay got the revelation to start a multimillion dollar cosmetic company when most people considered her ready for retirement. What they all had in common was that they surrounded themselves with the best, most creative, positive people they could find, and in that fertile ground, planted the seed of a great idea. When you have the benefit of one or more resourceful minds working on your idea, that idea is catapulted to a whole new realm of potential by way of the Infinite Intelligence. You can't do it alone!

Henry Ford admittedly did not have the answers to many of the questions that were asked of him concerning his business, or the world in general, for that matter. People assumed he was either a genius who should know everything, or an uneducated lucky guy who was in the right place at the right time and should be exposed as the fraud they believed him to be. In reality, he was neither of these extremes. Although lacking in extensive formal education, he took great pride in being able to find answers to questions people asked of him by consulting the experts he had rallied to be part of his Master Mind Alliance. From his desk, he could contact some of the most brilliant minds of the time and access their specialized knowledge. His success had much more to do with his ability to network than with anything his alleged genius or limited classroom experience may have given him. By his own admission, the success of the entire Ford Motor Company was a manifestation of the great minds with which he surrounded himself. This ability, combined with incredible diligence, more than made up for his lack of formal education.

You will never know the answer to every question asked concerning health and fitness. What is more important is your ability to find answers, and that involves having access to your own personal knowledge pool and tapping it on a regular basis. Surround yourself with brilliant minds in your field and watch how fast your mind expands to reach higher levels. In our profession, some of the people you should consider aligning yourself with are other successful trainers, physical therapists, medical doctors, chiropractors, nurses, mental therapists, aerobic instructors, school coaches, people in the ski industry, sport teammates, and karate people, just to name a few. The most obvious advantage, but certainly not the only one, of being in a group such as this is that its members can refer clients to one another.

I have a friend who is making a very lucrative income exclusively training the patients of a busy physical therapy clinic. She got the job by giving a soggy business card to one of the therapists in a sauna at her health club and offering her a free training session. Once the therapist was sold, she persuaded a few of her partners to train with my friend. They started sending her their clients, and before she knew it, she was booked. All because of one soggy business card and a free session! Since all her referrals are coming from therapists, and exercise is considered a legitimate and important part of most rehab treatment, insurance picks up the bulk of the tab. Ironically, many of these clients have chosen to continue training with my friend long after the insurance money has dried up, due to the fact that she's such a wonderful trainer.

The quality and quantity of your clientele are direct reflections of how you see yourself, how others see you, and the type of people with whom you've chosen to surround yourself. If you don't currently like where you are in this business, chances are you need to strengthen one of these areas of your life, and there is no time like the present to make the kind of changes that will turn the whole thing around.

In the past, I have doubled my income in less than a year due to the simple fact that I changed the way I was thinking, took on new allies, and positioned myself in a higher-visibility situation. You, too, have the power to start seeing success as a trainer, but it involves taking these first steps. I know this from personal experience.

Summary

🏃 *Know what your resources are: your body/mind balance, your ability to get high-end exposure, and the people in your network.*

🏃 *Establish and apply these resources to your business.*

🏃 *Develop the ability to take clients through vanity and bring them to real self-confidence. (Help your clients to reach a healthy balance.)*

🏃 *Be aware of the role vanity plays in your own life as well as in the lives of your clients.*

🏃 *Position yourself in such a way as to get maximum visual exposure. (Start by getting a job at a high-end, popular facility.)*

🏃 *Stay busy training people. (If you have no clients, bring in friends, family, and coworkers.)*

🏃 *Carefully pick the people you'll have in your "Master Mind Alliance." (This is the best means to get support and enhances your ability to network.)*

🏃 *Treat everyone who asks you about fitness as though he or she were the President.*

🏃 *Know that the quality and quantity of your clientele—or lack of one—is a direct reflection of how you've been thinking, where you've positioned yourself, and the type of people you've chosen to surround yourself with in the past. (Always look at these three areas if you're not happy with the results you're seeing in your business.)*

6

Educating Our Clients

*A*n issue that consistently seems to come up for us as trainers is that the majority of the people we train have a limited understanding of why and how diet and exercise work on their bodies. Since you are their primary source of fitness information, clients will inevitably come to you with questions concerning anatomy, physiology, kinesiology, resistance training, aerobics, health, diet, and metabolism. Not only do you need to know the answers to their questions, but you must also develop the ability to communicate these answers in ways that provide the client a reasonable understanding. The ability to take complex physiological concepts and accurately net out simple explanations that the average lay person can understand is an invaluable skill that is often overlooked when trainers develop their exercise systems.

Of all the reasons that educating our clients about their bodies is important, perhaps the most significant one is that it eliminates the ignorance excuse that many of them had been using to justify not taking responsibility for their health in the past. What you are in essence doing is giving them a legitimate reprieve by saying, "Hey, you didn't know this stuff before, but now you do because I'm telling you, and, from here on out, our goal is to take this knowledge and move forward into a healthier future. Are you committed, or not?" This approach allows them to take responsibility for their present and future health, without feeling really bad about screwing up in the past.

Educating your clients should be an ongoing process that is included in every training session you do. The more knowledge they have about their bodies, the more apt they'll be to stick with you and your program. Understanding the different ways a person's metabolism changes as he or she gets older, for instance, will give your clients more incentive to participate in some form of exercise routine well into their later years. When you clearly explain the changes their bodies are going through and will encounter, as well as how exercise will affect those changes, you'll be giving them the best reason in the world to continue exercising even after they've reached their short-term goals. The knowledge you give your clients will also help to sustain them through those periods when exercising may not be their biggest priority.

By describing, for example, why leg muscles function seventy-five percent more efficiently when they burn fat as opposed to sugar, you'll help them to visualize the process of losing weight as their bodies burn this fuel. When they know where major muscle groups are located and what their basic functions are, they'll gain a better understanding of how muscles support each other when the body lifts or pulls things, for example (biceps, lats, hamstrings, and erectors), or how it pushes things away (triceps, pecs, deltoids, and abs). Taking the time to give your clients a firm foundation of knowledge about their anatomies, which they'll be able to ingest in moderate doses over an extended period, will add "teacher" to the list of titles with which you'll be associated.

Not only is it important to teach your clients how and why their bodies function the way they do, but it is also essential to explain how your system of exercise will help them function more efficiently. Introducing them to exercises that are enjoyable, challenging, and varied, in combination with their newfound knowledge, will give them the confidence to explore whole new worlds of physical potential that they may not have been aware existed. The challenge you'll face is in conveying this knowledge without overwhelming them.

At the beginning of my career, I took pride in my ability to answer most questions my clients had about their bodies using the type of scientific terminology only a second-year medical student could appreciate. I loved quoting the latest studies, data, opinions, and theories of some of the greatest minds in the fitness world (at least in their estimation), and I mistakenly believed clients would be impressed if I answered their questions using every technical term I'd ever heard. Around that time, I learned another valuable lesson.

During his workout one morning, a client brought up the topic of spot reduction after finishing a set of crunches. I said I didn't believe it was possible, and he asked me why, which led to a discussion about how fat really is burned. Feeling exceptionally filled with knowledge that day, I proceeded to lay down my fat-burning rap with the kind of scientific abandon that would make even Einstein slap his knee and give me a hearty thumbs-up. The words began to flow so fast that in a matter of minutes I had the poor guy submerged in a sea of metabolic terminology that even I couldn't navigate.

Finally, in the middle of a sentence, he stopped me and said, "Ed, although I'm quite impressed with your understanding of metabolic concepts, to be honest, I can't follow a damn thing you're saying! I have two degrees and still can't make sense out of all the sciento-babble you're trying to impress me with, so please, if spot reduction doesn't work, simply tell me in layman's terms how the other stuff you're having me do is going to help me get rid of my gut!"

That little chastising was actually very helpful in that it allowed me to realize two of the most important things that all clients need to feel when they are with us. Those two things are a sense of empowerment and a clear understanding of how exercise works with their bodies. What my client needed when he asked me about his fat was not only the hope that I could help him reduce it, but the clarity to explain why. He needed to feel that all the work I was having him do was for a reason and to understand why every diet or program he had tried in the past hadn't worked. What I gave him was a batch of confusing terms that only served to make him feel more frustrated and defensive, and ultimately stifled our line of communication.

The Seat of Power

Think of the process of empowering clients as a three-legged stool, with the legs representing three different modes of empowerment. The first leg represents physical empowerment, which is obviously achieved through your exercise program. The second is emotional empowerment, which is achieved through your ability to motivate your clients to establish and maintain the drive needed to reach their goals. The third leg is mental empowerment, which is your ability to clearly and logically explain the changes their bodies will be going through as they continue to exercise. If you remove any of the three legs from the stool, it falls over.

I was great at creating exercise programs and motivating clients, but I didn't offer a complete fitness package until I developed the ability to educate them as well. When people have questions concerning their bodies, quite often they're already coming from a place of confusion and misinformation. If you baffle them further with your explanation, they may lose enthusiasm or trust, and you may lose them. What clients look to you for is clarity.

Most people have at least a curiosity about how their bodies work, but don't want to seem ignorant about what little knowledge they may have on the subject. In the case of new, unfit clients, who may already feel less than wise for letting themselves get so out of shape, knowledge of their body holds a special importance in that it empowers them to abandon the misconceptions and fears that may have caused them to feel helpless in the past. A trainer's ability to simply, yet thoroughly, answer his or her clients' questions will place that person in higher demand than the trainer who either overkills an explanation or, on the other extreme, doesn't think educating clients is all that important. It's a balance.

Inevitably, you'll notice the same types of questions will keep coming up if you train people long enough, and my goal in this chapter is to answer what I've experienced to be the most commonly asked ones. Undoubtedly, some questions will come up that I haven't addressed; these can be answered by referencing the collateral material I'll recommend later on.

Here are the questions I've been asked most frequently:

🏃 *What is metabolism and how is it affected by exercise?*

🏃 *What types of activities will make a person's metabolism work more efficiently, and what steps can be taken to maintain its efficiency?*

🏃 *What are the benefits of aerobic versus anaerobic activity?*

🏃 *What are the benefits of strength and resistance training?*

🏃 *Why is muscle so important, and what is the best way to build it?*

🏃 *What is fat and what is it good for? What is the best way to burn it?*

🏃 *What is sugar and what does it do? Why is it easier to burn than fat?*

🏃 *What is ATP and how does it relate to metabolism?*

🏃 *What should one know about diet and how it fits into the picture?*

Metabolism Made Fun

This section will help you develop accurate yet simple answers to questions your clients may have concerning metabolism and how it relates to fitness training. I try to use language my clients can understand, instead of the dry scientific data that made some of us fall asleep in eleventh-grade anatomy class.

The subject of human metabolism is so vast it would take a lifetime for any one individual to master it. Although no one expects us to know it all, it is in our best interest as quality trainers to thoroughly understand and be able to communicate, at the very least, the aspect of metabolism that relates most closely to what we do. That aspect is "caloric" metabolism.

Clients will find a million different ways to ask the same few basic questions when it comes to this topic. Whether they're in great shape wanting to improve in a sport or in poor shape wanting to start a basic program, what they'll all want to know at some point or another is what role exercise plays in metabolizing calories and how this process impacts the way they eat, sleep, work, play, relax, do sports, and stress out.

You don't need to be a physician to answer most of the questions your clients will ask concerning food intake and exercise, but you do need a solid understanding of how calories are burned and/or stored if you wish to communicate even the basics of fitness to them. As much as possible, I try to make my answers easy to remember by using analogies and stories that are simple, not hard to understand, and I hope, fun to listen to.

If you're training people's bodies to be more fit, I trust, for the sake of our profession, that you already have knowledge of the concepts that I'm about to discuss. For trainers who know the concepts but find it difficult getting their clients to understand them, this section should be used as a review with an applicable twist. If you're a trainer who has little idea scientifically how muscle is built, or fat is burned off, for example, then read and learn before you give someone the wrong advice.

I highly recommend Covert Bailey's book, *Smart Exercise,* as a great source for collateral reading available on the subjects of physiology and exercise and how they relate to training and overall fitness. Bailey is the master at taking heavy science and making it user-friendly. Again, it's not a matter just of having the knowledge, of but being able to get it across to your clients. With that in mind, let's jump into science class and have some fun. (Can you spell "oxymoron"?)

Metabolism

Metabolism literally refers to every chemical reaction that takes place in the human body. When considering the multitude of different reactions that are involved, it's no wonder this subject has so many different categories, each with its own group of experts to explain their particular aspect to you. In the same hospital cafeteria, you'll find brain surgeons at one table discussing metabolism in concepts and terms vastly different from those used by the podiatrists or dietitians sitting at other tables. For this reason, it's ludicrous to think that any one individual could be an expert in it all, and you should be leery of people who imply they are.

The majority of your clients who want to understand metabolism really want to understand how their bodies burn calories, or more specifically, how they can burn off excess fat and gain muscle definition through exercise. When talking to clients about metabolism, they'll inevitably ask this question in some form: Why, as I get older, do I seem to gain more weight when I eat the same amount of food I've always eaten?

In order to address the answer to this question, you must first be able to explain in simple lay terms the nature of fat, glucose, protein, enzymes, insulin, glucagon, and ATP, and describe what their functions are (all in one breath!). By having knowledge of these seven substances individually, I find it easier to relate to clients how they come together in the big picture known as caloric metabolism.

In the beginning, there was:

Fat

When explaining fat to my clients, I first make sure they understand these four important facts:

1 The body's primary source of fuel is free fatty acids. They are found either stored in fat cells or surfing the bloodstream looking for muscles that need to burn them for energy.

2 Your body—more specifically, your liver—has the ability to take any food you eat, in excess of what it needs, and turn it into some form of fat.

3 No matter how out of shape a person is, his or her body can be taught to metabolize fatty acids more efficiently. The results are better health, weight loss, more energy, and a longer life.

4 Exercise, primarily aerobic in combination with resistance training, is the only practical way of teaching your body to burn fat and build muscle more efficiently.

What Is Fat?

The body has the ability to transform the food we eat into many different forms of fat. Some food will become **free fatty acids,** the circulating form of fat found in blood, which is primarily used for energy. Some will become **low- or high-density cholesterol,** and some will become **mono-, di-, or triglycerides.** Triglycerides are the body's primary storage form of fat. Think of them as individual glucose molecules that have been bound together in bundles of three for the purpose of being stored in fat cells. When clients ask me why their doctor needed to check their triglyceride level, I tell them that their fat cells became so packed with fat that some of it squirted back out into their bloodstream. The doctor was simply checking to see how much. Since triglycerides don't even belong in the bloodstream, a high level is often grounds for major diet and lifestyle changes. Refined sugar, alcohol, and high-fructose corn syrup are just a few of the things that exacerbate higher triglyceride levels.

These last five categories of fat make up the bulk of the fat that can be found in the bloodstream; they tend to either sit dormant or build up on the walls of arteries, increasing the risk of heart attack and stroke. Fatty acids, on the other hand, don't build up on artery walls. If they're not being burned, they can be found relaxing in fat cells.

As Covert Bailey describes it:

> Fatty acid molecules are extremely small compared to triglycerides and cholesterol—and they are highly mobile. It is easy for fatty acids to pass through semi-permeable membranes, the porous walls of capillaries and cells. They can move out of the bloodstream into a muscle cell to be burned for energy. If the muscle cell says, "I'm not exercising right now," they move back out into the blood again and travel to a fat cell for storage.

The average person is confused on the subject of fat, most likely due to the multitude of different names associated with it. A biochemist, for example, would probably call cholesterol a lipid, and a pathologist would most likely refer to stored triglycerides as adipose tissue. Most people tend to call all of the categories just plain old fat, which is where a lot of misconceptions begin.

Again, your goal is to keep your answers as simple and informative as possible. Don't get so caught up in your terminology that you lose sight of your basic explanation. Your clients will show much more interest in knowing how exercise will help burn off the fatty acids stored in their tummy tire than in understanding the molecular structure of linoleic acid and how it helps to synthesize prostaglandin. More on fat later.

Glucose (The Other Fuel)

All carbohydrates and sugars (simple or complex), when ingested by the body, are turned into blood glucose, or blood sugar. It is directly used as an energy source for certain tissue such as the brain and retina. In excess, it's stored either as glycogen in muscle or liver cells or as triglycerides in fat cells.

The term glycogen refers to a row or chain of glucose molecules that have been strung together for the purpose of being stored, specifically, in muscle and liver cells. These molecules are broken off and used one at a time by active muscles until the chain runs out, at which time the muscles must either start burning fat, or rest and replenish their spent glycogen if they wish to continue the activity. The problem with replacing spent glycogen is that it can only be restrung and stored at a rate of five percent an hour, regardless of how much the person eats or rests. This rate is slightly higher for the first two hours after an anaerobic activity, after which time it slows back down to the five percent rebuilding rate. Simply put: The body burns glycogen when short bursts of intense muscular energy are needed; stored free fatty acids, on the other hand, are used when sustained, long-distance muscular energy is required.

Unlike stored free fatty acids, which make their home in fat cells and involve a delicate balance of oxygen and specialized enzymes in order to be tapped for energy, glycogen is stored in muscle and liver cells. It can be tapped at a moment's notice, with or without oxygen, using some of the most basic enzymes the liver can produce. Glycogen allows the body to rally a small amount of energy fast (the flight or fight mechanism). The downside of this is that it burns up so quickly that it can't be counted on to supply any kind of sustained energy.

Where muscles are concerned, another, perhaps more important, function of glycogen is that it acts as a kind of kindling for the fat-burning fire to take place. This is where the real energy lies. Without a little half-burned sugar to stoke it, the fat fire goes out, along with any energy it may have been producing. Later in this chapter, I'll discuss in detail how sugar and fat are actually burned.

Insulin/Glucagon

Apart from diabetic clients or clients in medical professions, I find most of the general public to be surprisingly ignorant of the functions of the pancreas. Everyone knows what the heart and kidneys do. Most people seem to have a basic sense of how the lungs and liver work. But just ask the average person on the street what the pancreas does and you'll likely get a blank stare. For this reason, when the discussion of metabolism turns to the topic of blood sugar, I always find that I have to do a little remedial work. Most clients need a basic understanding of what the pancreas does. It puts things into a clearer perspective.

I explain that there are numerous reasons a body must maintain a delicate balance of blood glucose, but by far the most important one is to keep the brain alive and happy. All other biological functions can be plugging along just fine, but when the brain shuts down, all the fun goes out of life. For this reason, the body will literally sacrifice its own muscle tissue if it means finding enough nutrients to keep the brain alive.

Most tissue in the body can survive using glycogen, fat, or even protein as fuel, but brain tissue is temperamental and only functions when just the right amount of pure, unaltered glucose is present. Whereas other areas of the body can easily adjust to varying levels of glucose, the brain quickly chokes on either too much or too little. (If a body's blood sugar level goes below a critical point, the brain starves. If the level goes above a certain point, the brain becomes poisoned.)

When glucose levels are too high, the excess spills out of the blood and into the urine, pulling with it large amounts of water to help dilute and flush the system as quickly as possible. This is the body's last-ditch effort to lower its glucose concentration. It explains why diabetics who aren't consistent with their maintenance program often experience severe thirst and at the same time have to pee a lot. When one considers the many different functions that water serves in keeping a body alive, it becomes apparent that this most important commodity cannot be disproportionately monopolized for the purpose of eliminating toxins. When too much water is used for the removal of toxins, other bodily functions pay a high price. The most extreme price to be paid is that the transportation of oxygen to, you guessed it, the brain becomes compromised. When the body becomes critically dehydrated and can't oxygenate its brain cells, the brain starves. The next stages are coma and death.

At this point, you're probably asking, "If there is excess sugar in the blood, can't your body just burn it off or store it in fat cells? If it runs low, can't your body break down fat or protein and use them as fuel to make up the difference?" Good questions!

The bottom line is, when the brain experiences either an overdose or a shortage of blood sugar, all systems of the body go on red alert and work together to reestablish the delicate balance needed to maintain its function. Just a few minutes of critically low blood glucose is enough to cause the brain to shut down. The problem is, none of the body's systems can process glucose fast enough to maintain the needed balance.

Insulin and glucagon to the rescue!

These guys are hormones secreted by the pancreas, whose job it is to quickly lower or heighten the blood's glucose level. The secreted amount of either one is in direct proportion to how high or low the blood sugar level is at any given time. How do they work?

Let's make believe you just finished eating an Italian meal that included lots of pasta and bread. Although pasta and bread are considered complex carbohydrates, the fact that they are heavily refined, therefore quickly digested, causes them to turn into blood sugar almost as fast as they hit your stomach. As your blood glucose level rises to a hyper-glycemic state, an alarm goes off and your pancreas gets the signal to secrete insulin. The insulin proceeds to usher the excess glucose out of your bloodstream and encourages it to be stored in your fat, muscle, and liver cells in the form of either triglycerides or glycogen, thus lowering the amount in the blood.

Now, let's pretend you're three to four hours into a beautiful mountain hike. After doing a little hand jive in your day pack, you realize you've left your lunch on the kitchen counter. As your glucose level goes down, you'll begin to feel tired and light-headed. As your energy level continues to drop, a lower-sounding alarm goes off and signals the other side of your pancreas to secrete glucagon. This miracle hormone has the ability to take the remaining glycogen from your liver and muscle cells, tap the fatty acids from your fat cells, and turn them back into individual glucose molecules that make their way back into your bloodstream to feed your brain and give you enough energy to make it back home to your fridge.

Just remember, hyperglycemia, or high blood sugar, stimulates the secretion of insulin, which takes sugar out of blood cells and puts it into other cells. Hypoglycemia, or low blood sugar, stimulates the secretion of glucagon, which breaks down cellular glycogen and fat into basic glucose and puts it back into blood.

"Okay, Ed," I hear you say. "How often am I going to talk to one of my clients about hormones and insulin, and what do they have to do with fit-ness training anyway?" Boy, you are tough!

Another Story

One day I was having a discussion with a moderately overweight woman who had recently allowed herself to get out of shape. As we talked about nutrition and exercise, the conversation drifted to the subject of hunger and big muscles. She wanted to know why she always felt the craving for more food an hour or so after a meal and why every time she tried lifting weights, even lightly, she'd rapidly gain weight and get even hungrier. "Isn't light weightlifting supposed to give you muscle definition and curb your hunger?" she asked. On those rare occasions when she did anything aerobic like distance walking or hiking, she'd be ravenous right afterward, which caused her to eat even more than she did when she lifted weights. It seemed everything this woman did made her hungry. (Although she was eating all the time, to look at her, you wouldn't really say she was fat. I'd describe her more as big.) Only a few years earlier, she had been lean, athletic, active in several different sports, and dedicated to working out in some way every day.

Her current goal was to reestablish her lost muscle definition while getting rid of the fifteen pounds of fat she had gained over the last three years. Her plan was to do it by eating only oatmeal with fruit for breakfast and rice or pasta with vegetables for dinner, and working out with me twice a week.

Somewhere, several years ago, she had read that eating sugar and fat was bad, but carbohydrates were okay as long as you did some form of exercise. This gave her the inspiration to eat carbohydrates with total abandon and justify it because she didn't think they were fats or sugar. Plus, she was active and did some exercise, which she thought would burn off any excess.

Although she considered herself active, her current activities were of a different type than when she was an athlete. The truth was, almost all the activities at that point in her life were anaerobic in nature, which didn't allow her to burn the kind of fat she needed to reach her goal. (In her glory days, most of the activities she did were aerobic.) On top of that, the fact that she had given up all exercise for a few years caused her body to naturally metabolize food more for storage and less for fuel.

I knew that her mostly-carbohydrate diet, plus the kind of exercise she wanted to do (light weight-training with minimal aerobic activity), wouldn't give her the kind of fat loss or muscle definition she was expecting, because her body would still be storing more fat than it was burning. By describing what was going on with her body in hormonal terms, I was able to explain why she was always hungry and had trouble losing the weight.

I explained to her that all the carbohydrates she ate were quickly being turned into glucose, which would inevitably stimulate the secretion of higher levels of insulin. Without the benefit of aerobic exercise, the insulin was encouraging her body to store sugar and fat, and at the same time inhibiting her body's ability to release them for fuel. Her constant hunger was a manifestation of her body's inability to heighten its blood sugar level using its own storehouses. This was due to her pancreas producing too much insulin.

How ironic! Insulin, produced to help lower her blood sugar, would actually lower it to the point that she always felt hungry and had to eat more in order to get it higher. The higher level would in turn produce more insulin, which would decrease her glucose level, ultimately increasing her hunger and ability to store fat, but not burn it. Barry Sears, author of *The Zone*, says:

> The craving that comes 90 minutes after a huge pasta meal means that the insulin has carried the glucose away and that it's preventing your body from getting at the glycogen that's stored in your liver. Your sugar starved brain is telling you to turn to external resources for more. You're entering carbohydrate hell—you're a slave to Oreos.

What advice did I give this client? First, I convinced her that exercise consisting of sporadic anaerobic activities (light resistance training once or twice a week with minimal aerobic exertion), combined with the type of food she was eating, would only serve to make her bigger and hungrier. Since she wasn't doing significant aerobic exercise, her body wasn't forced to burn major sugar and carbohydrate calories; instead, after becoming glucose, these only served to make more insulin and pack her fat cells. When she combined high carbohydrates with sporadic anaerobic activities like weightlifting, what she got were undefined muscles covered with fat, and a constant hunger for more carbohydrates.

I knew that buried just beneath the surface, she had what once were strong, defined muscles with memory, and my intent was to wake them up and maintain them. The fact that she was strong led me to believe that her muscles were still in fair shape, which meant that we could concentrate our efforts on burning the fat around them as we redeveloped their definition. I designed her program aerobically to include power walking, riding her bike, or using her Nordic Track without stopping for at least one hour four times a week. To bring back her definition, we incorporated medium to heavy free weights with lots of repetitions three times per week.

A concern she had was that her muscles were already too big and they didn't even look like muscles. They were covered with just enough fat to make her look big, but not defined. Muscles covered and marbled with fat tend to look like, well, fat muscles, not the lean ones of her active days. Her fear was that by increasing her resistance training both in weights and duration, she'd get even bigger and hungrier. I explained that this program would do the exact opposite. By combining mostly aerobic exercise with three hard days of weight training, she would actually lose fat and increase definition without getting bigger, although she might only drop five pounds of scale weight. The more muscles she developed, the more fat she'd have to burn to maintain them. Her hunger would subside because the aerobic training she agreed to do would put demands on her system to burn more glycogen for fuel, instead of having it produce more insulin to store fuel. When her blood sugar did spike, she'd need less insulin to lower it because more glucose would naturally be pulled out and used to rebuild the glycogen she had depleted while doing her aerobics. In reality, she didn't care how much she weighed as long as she didn't look so big. She had a preconceived idea that her size was mostly due to her muscles getting bigger, but after doing a fat caliber test, we were both surprised to see she had around 28% body fat. (Both of us guessed she would have had around 22%.)

Her body, like those of most people who were once athletic and muscular but have allowed themselves to become flabby, seemed to get huge with just a little bit of weight training, which caused her to blame the weights instead of looking at the real culprit. She was trying to get in shape by using the training techniques she used when she was younger and much more athletic. What she failed to remember was that she also used to run and bike for long distances, which caused her to burn all sorts of fatty acids that she wasn't burning at present. As for her diet, I had her cut back her carbohydrate intake to one-third of every meal and to eat the other two-thirds as protein. The plan was to eat five smaller meals a day using this one-to-two-parts combination. Simple, yet very effective.

Three months after beginning the program, this woman's body went through some profound visual changes. As predicted, she only lost about eight pounds, but the beauty was that it was all fat. How do we know it was all fat? Because we were building her muscles the whole time and they looked great. She went down one full waist size, and to look at her you'd think she'd lost eighteen pounds instead of eight. Almost as an afterthought, she realized she wasn't hungry twenty hours a day, which made her feel that she had more control of her life. By changing just a few elements of her eating and workout habits, she went from spinning her sugar wheels in the mud to burning her stored fat fuel all-out on the open road.

Trainer's Note: It has been my experience that, when talking to clients about caloric metabolism, some, especially ex-athletes like this woman, seem to respond better if I describe things in hormonal terms. In contrast, those clients who have never been in great shape seem to respond better when I describe metabolism using terms relating to enzymes, which I talk about later in the chapter on enzymes. I have no idea why these two groups would respond more to one description than the other, but they do. Try varying your explanations and see how your clients respond.

Protein

As we've been taught, all the protein we ingest breaks down into its main component, amino acids. The liver has the unique ability to take these amino acids and change their shape and form into any number of different enzymes, or "tools," which the body may use to perform specific tasks. When the tasks are completed and that particular tool is no longer needed, the same protein can be changed back into amino acids or reshaped into another tool, which can then be used to perform yet another task. Enzymes are constantly changing shape to accommodate the different demands of the body, and their origin is always amino acids. Here is one of the visual analogies that I use with my clients to get the point across.

Imagine a small troupe of actors and actresses (protein), who have taken on the task of performing a large production that involves many diverse characters, like *Romeo and Juliet*. Because there are more characters than actors to play them, each actor may need to play more than one part in order to complete the production. The director (the body) may point to one actor and say, "I need you to play the hot-blooded Mercutio in Act Three, Scene One, and I also need you to play Friar John in Act Five, Scene Two." An actress may be called upon to play Lady Montague in one scene and Juliet's nurse in another. In order to pull this off, the actors must run backstage after each scene and, with the help of the makeup artist (the liver), transform into entirely new characters.

Let's take this analogy one step further to show how versatile protein can be. One of my favorite clients, Neil, is the orchestra conductor for the Boulder Dinner Theater. At every show I've had the pleasure of attending, I'm always impressed at how many different roles the production cast and Neil take in the course of the evening. First, the cast assumes the role of waiters and waitresses by taking your dinner order, serving you drinks, and bringing your food. The next thing you know, those same people are up on stage, acting, singing, and dancing their hearts out. At intermission, they're back clearing plates and serving dessert. Then, it's up on stage again to finish the play. Neil not only conducts the orchestra, but also tends bar and somehow always finds time to come and sit at my table at intermission, which makes me look good if I have a date. At the end of the evening, the cast could, hypothetically, be asked to stay late and fix any broken furniture, in case the audience got out of hand.

The crew at the dinner theater are just like the amino acids in protein. They can be turned into any number of different turbochargers the body needs to speed up its numerous functions, and they can even be used as substitute nutrients when the body can't find them anywhere else. In the absence of carbohydrates, for example, amino acids can be turned into something similar to a glucose molecule, which, in a pinch, can be substituted for the sugar that feeds the brain and kindles the fat-burning fire.

Although protein can be used in many ways, it has two primary functions in the body. It is essential for the growth and repair of tissue, and it is also converted into different types of enzymes. Using protein in any other way is not using it efficiently. To use it as fuel, for example, may cause other areas of the body, which may be protein dependent, to suffer. As Bailey puts it, "It doesn't seem right to use amino acids intended for tissue repair simply as a fuel. That's as silly as burning expensive two-by-fours in your fireplace instead of a cheaper, more easily available fuel."

Enzymes

When discussing enzymes with my clients, I first make sure they understand the basic nature of protein. I explain that enzymes are made out of amino acids, which started out as protein. Their purpose is to speed up specific bodily functions, and when that job is completed, they can be turned back into amino acids, which can then be reshaped again into other enzymes to be used to help perform other tasks.

Without enzymes, the metabolic and chemical reactions taking place in the human body would simply take too long to provide the growth, energy, repair, and maintenance the body needs to function. Simply put, enzymes are proteins designed to speed up the rate at which metabolic reactions occur. Some reactions that would take hours or even days to happen under normal laboratory conditions can take place in seconds under the influence of enzymes in the body. Physiology books refer to them as biological catalysts, but I like to think of them as something akin to a turbocharger on a sports car.

One of the many functions of the liver is to turn amino acids into different types of enzymes to be used as the body needs them. These amino acids are stored in pools that are located throughout the body in muscle tissue, in the liver, and even in blood. When you ingest a large meal, some of those amino acids are turned into digestion enzymes, which are used in conjunction with stomach acids to break down the food. If you were crazy enough to want to run a wind-sprint, after an hour or so, some of those leftover, recycled amino acids could be turned into sugar-burning enzymes that your body would require to burn the glycogen you would need to run full blast for a short period of time.

As a trainer, the three types of enzymes you'll need to be most familiar with are: sugar-burning enzymes, fat-burning enzymes, and Krebs Cycle enzymes. When talking to clients about anything from weight loss to physical endurance, I find it helpful to include a description of how these separate sets of enzymes work. I tell them that within each muscle cell of a healthy body, a three-stage fuel-burning process takes place in order to create the energy the muscle needs to do its job. An unhealthy body may only have the capacity to use the first and second stages. Each stage of burning requires its own unique set of enzymes in order to take place. The first stage, sugar-burning, can take place with or without oxygen. The next two stages, fat-burning and the Krebs Cycle, can only take place aerobically, when oxygen is present. Stage one and stage two require that glycogen and fatty acids be broken down halfway into a substance called pyruvic acid. The third stage of burning, or what's referred to as the Krebs Cycle, involves burning pyruvic acid down to carbon dioxide and water. (Pyruvic acid will be discussed in the section on The Krebs Cycle.)

1 Sugar-Burning Enzymes

The body's need to consistently burn glycogen and glucose, whether it is strenuously exercising or sitting on the couch eating ice cream, make it necessary to have an abundance of sugar-burning enzymes on hand at all times. These guys are quite stable and, as mentioned earlier, can burn sugar either aerobically or anaerobically. They do not disappear if you don't exercise and are ready to go to work burning sugar at a moment's notice. By not exercising, inactive, unfit, or overweight people tend to become dependent upon sugar-burning enzymes and the glycogen they burn. Since their bodies don't burn significant amounts of fat, their level of energy is in direct proportion to the limited amount of glycogen that has been stored in their muscle cells at any given time. When that sugar is burned up, so is their energy. Because they lack fat-burning enzymes, maintain poor VO_2 max ratings, very rarely leave their anaerobic state due to difficulty in moving their bulk, and have limited glycogen stores, it's no wonder unfit people run out of steam so fast. The human body has the ability to store massive amounts of fat, but without the right enzymes to access it, it just sits in the old fuel tank waiting to be burned.

Since sugar-burning enzymes are always present whether the person exercises or not, it's easy to see how an unfit body may become solely dependent on the sugar system as its main source of energy. This works great as long as the body isn't called upon to do anything more physical than eating or walking across the street. At a certain point, the body, in a sense, forgets how to burn fat and starts to believe that sugar burning is all that's needed to get through life. (Talk about metabolic denial!)

Consistent aerobic exercise decreases the body's dependency on the sugar-burning system by multiplying its fat-burning enzymes, thus giving it the ability to burn more fat. In contrast, lack of exercise diminishes the body's capacity to generate these enzymes, which explains why unfit people tend to store more fat than they burn. Remember: asking a body to function efficiently using only sugar as fuel is like trying to drive a car from Denver to Kansas City using only first gear, with a fuel tank that only holds two gallons of gas. Good luck!

2 Fat-Burning Enzymes

Think of fat-burning enzymes as a specialized group of highly trained gladiators during Roman times.

If the Coliseum had only a few cheap seat ticket holders in it, like on Monday or Tuesday night, you could just imagine Caesar ordering a few peasants (sugar-burning enzymes) to be eaten by lions instead of using gladiatorial entertainment to appease such a small weekday crowd. Gladiator contests were done only on Friday and Saturday nights, when the place was jammin' and the crowd was serious. On really busy nights, peasants were also used to warm up the crowd for the main event.

Unlike peasants, whose numbers were vast and who didn't have a lot of crowd-pleasing talent (how much talent does it take to be eaten by a lion?), gladiators were in limited supply and had great value due to their incredible fighting abilities and crowd-pleasing skills. The time and energy that went into training them to be great fighters made them an asset to Caesar, and their talents were never wasted. For this reason, they were pampered. They always got the best food and accommodations, and they didn't have to fight unless the house was packed and the air in the coliseum was clean and full of oxygen. They'd whine that without enough oxygen, they would get headaches and couldn't fight. (This may be where the phrase, "Not tonight, I have a headache," came from.)

In order for gladiators to do their job well, they had to stay in top physical shape by exercising and competing on a regular basis. When, for whatever reason, gladiators couldn't consistently compete, they'd get lazy, and some would drop out of the profession entirely and become Roman senators.

Fat-burning enzymes are just like those strong, charming, temperamental Roman gladiators. They don't go to work unless the body is serious and the conditions are just right, and this includes having lots of oxygen. They are called to action when a fit body is pushed beyond its ability to sustain its current level of activity due to its glycogen stores running low. Because fit bodies have the ability to generate fat-burning enzymes, they can easily go from sugar-burning to fat-burning in their quest for more sustainable fuel.

An unfit body can't make the transition, not for lack of stored fuel, but for lack of enzymes to help burn the fuel. For an unfit person to continue doing any lengthy physical activity, he or she must periodically stop, sit down, and wait for more sugar to trickle into his or her muscle cells in order to finish whatever it was he or she was doing. Fit people don't need to stop; they just shift into a higher gear.

3 Krebs Cycle Enzymes

If the first stages of sugar and fat burning are like discovering small veins of gold in a gold mine, the Krebs Cycle is like striking the mother lode.

As mentioned earlier, sugar and fat are half-burned down to a substance known as pyruvic acid. (I just had an image of thousands of clients across the country asking their personal trainers in unison, "What is pyruvic acid?")

If you've ever tried making home-brewed beer, you must have encountered a nasty substance called mash, or what I like to refer to as "stinky mash." It's a combination of sugar, grain, hops, fruit, and water that has been smashed together and left to ferment for a period of time. The goal of a good home brewmaster is to take this bubbly, fermented, weird-smelling soup and, by adding yeast at just the right time, process it down to alcoholic brew.

The environmental conditions have to be just right in order for this final stage of breakdown to take place. If any elements are missing or the conditions aren't perfect, what you end up with is something that looks and smells as bad as, if not worse than, the original mashy stuff.

Pyruvic acid is like stinky mash. Think of it as sugar and fat that have been half-broken down into a substance that no longer looks like sugar or fat, but maintains some of the characteristics of both.

When Krebs Cycle enzymes are available to break down pyruvic acid, what results is an enormous amount of pure, unstoppable physical energy. Muscles requiring this type of major sustained energy, as in most highly physical activities like racquetball, track, basketball, or soccer, must go to this higher source of power, this potentate of energy, this grand marshal of endurance—the Krebs Cycle—in order to obtain it.

In lay terms, the Krebs Cycle involves the burning of pyruvic acid down to carbon dioxide and water. The three elements that must be present to perform this task are:

🏃 *half-burned sugar and fat*

🏃 *Krebs Cycle enzymes, and*

🏃 *oxygen (a little unburned sugar is needed to ignite the fire).*

Unlike sugar and fat, which must enter a muscle cell from the outside to be burned inside, pyruvic acid is created inside the muscle cell, where it awaits oxygen and enzymes in order to ignite. The energy produced is like that of an oil-well fire, which burns with a hot, slow, and constant flame, as opposed to a gasoline fire, which explodes and then goes out. If pyruvic acid is burned off completely, all that is left is carbon dioxide, which is released out of the body through the breath, and water, which is either sweated out of the body or absorbed back into the system. If pyruvic acid is not burned off completely, what is left over becomes lactic acid, which causes the burning sensation in specific muscle groups. Normally this only occurs during workouts when muscles are isolated or when the body enters an anaerobic state. Remember, without oxygen, pyruvic acid and fat can't burn. This is why working more muscle groups together and

exercising them aerobically is more efficient than isolating them anaerobically, if the goal is to burn fat. When numerous muscle groups are
involved in an aerobic exercise, more pyruvic acid is burned, which means
more energy is produced and less lactic acid is created.

ATP (Adenosine Triphosphate)

Note: Before explaining ATP to your clients, keep in mind that it is a
fairly complex topic, not unlike metabolism, which can quickly get deep
and confusing if you let it get away from you. Remember, your goal is to
give your clients a simplified lesson in fitness as it relates to physiology
and anatomy without overwhelming them. Keep your explanations accurate yet simple, and your clients will love you for it. This is how I might
explain ATP to a client:

Ed: Okay, we've established that muscle cells burn sugar and fat down
to a halfway point, producing a moderate amount of energy. The
half-burned sugar then becomes kindling for the half-burned fat,
producing substantially more energy, as it is broken further down
into carbon dioxide and water. This stage (the Krebs Cycle) is
where the bulk of the energy is produced when a body does long-
term aerobic activity.

Client: I understand that, but how does that energy actually make my
muscles work?

Ed: The answer is, it doesn't. The energy produced by burning sugar
and fat is used to make a substance known as adenosine triphosphate (ATP). Every cell in the entire body functions with energy
produced by ATP, but it is active muscle cells that require the
most, due to the nature of their function. What happens is that a
little explosive charge takes place inside each ATP molecule, producing a spark of energy, which is then used to contract the
muscle. Active muscles always produce more ATP than the rest
of the body in order to work.

Client: Tell me about the explosive charge.

Ed: Imagine a bullet, consisting of a long shell casing filled with gunpowder (one molecule of adenosine) with a lead projectile sitting on top (three molecules of phosphorus or triphosphate.) Now, imagine the bullet being fired. At the moment the lead projectile becomes dislodged from the casing, a spark of energy occurs. That spark of energy, created by triphosphates separating themselves from the main molecule, is what causes muscles to contract. The power is in the separation. (Profound!) That fired projectile and spent casing can now be reused and made back into a whole new bullet, but energy is required to reconnect them. This involves calorie burning. The energy produced by burning fat and sugar is what the body uses to put the lead back on the casing.. Once the bullet is put back together, it can be exploded again and again provided there is enough energy to rebuild it.

Client: Give me an example of how my muscles might use the ATP energy.

Ed: After a long day of consistent, strenuous activity, muscle cells go on a mission to replenish their glycogen stores as quickly as possible. One example of how ATP works is that it produces the energy needed to bond single glucose molecules together to form new glycogen. A simple candy bar after a hard run will replenish most of the glucose the body has used, but muscle cells don't work with glucose; they need glycogen, and in order to produce it, ATP energy is needed.

Client: If ATP is needed to produce the energy to make glycogen, what happens when the activity is such that it wipes out not only the cell's glycogen but its ATP as well? In other words, how do you make glycogen when you've run out of ATP?

Ed: The answer is fat. When glycogen runs low, fat-burning supplies the energy to make the ATP, which supplies the energy needed to make more glycogen, which then helps burn more fat to complete the Krebs Cycle. (And around and around it goes.) Remember, fatty acids and half-burned fatty acids (in the Krebs Cycle) are the body's long-distance fuel that will never run out and can always be burned, as long as you have the right enzymes, oxygen, and a little half-burned sugar. When these three ingredients are present, fat can always be burned to create ATP.

Client: Why do even fit bodies have trouble sustaining wind sprints or similar anaerobic activity for any length of time, and how does ATP fit in?

Ed: During anaerobic activity, ATP can't be replaced as fast as it's used up. Since the body isn't using oxygen, it loses its ability to create ATP from its main fuel source, fat-burning. The only fuel that works during anaerobic activity is glycogen, but it can't produce ATP fast enough by itself to keep up with the demands of sprinting. When the body has depleted its stored ATP (needed to rebuild glycogen) and is lacking in oxygen (needed to burn fat), it virtually loses its ability to rebuild new ATP, which muscles need to contract. At that point, the body must ultimately stop and rest, or slow down to an aerobic state in order to let oxygen back in.

Client: Is ATP rebuilt during or after the activity?

Ed: As long as they breathe steadily, fit bodies rebuild ATP, not only during the activity, but also in the resting period afterwards. In order to replenish ATP as well as glycogen, major calorie-burning from fat is required. This explains why fit people continue to burn fat, even while resting, long after a hard workout. Unfit bodies don't burn significant calories replacing ATP and glycogen because they don't deplete significant amounts of them to begin with. You need to flex muscles in order to deplete glycogen. Since unfit bodies aren't good at making fat-burning enzymes, they don't burn a lot of fat. Most of their ATP energy must come from the calories produced by sugar-burning (anaerobic glycolysis), which is a cheap, unstable source at best.

Client: Does a person's level of fitness have anything to do with how fast ATP and glycogen are replaced in his or her body?

Ed: Yes, fit bodies are able to replace both of these substances up to fifty percent faster than unfit bodies. **Note:** At their best, fit bodies can still only replace their spent glycogen at a rate of five percent an hour. In unfit bodies, glucose isn't needed to make more glycogen, so it's carted off to be stored in fat cells. In fit bodies, glucose is needed, especially after a hard workout, to replace the glycogen that has been burned up during the activity. And ATP energy makes the whole thing happen.

If a client is still confused after this type of explanation, you can try another tack, which I'll explain in the next chapter.

7 *A Cautionary Tale*

*E*xperience has taught me that if I need my clients to remember something important about their bodies, it's best to explain it to them using some form of analogy, comparison, or funny story. I understand not everyone is good at telling stories or coming up with analogies, so I've included a few examples to get your imagination going. Nothing makes a lasting impression in a client's mind better than a story about two hypothetical people, one being quite healthy and the other being extremely unhealthy for contrast.

Once I've developed a clear profile of these two extremes, I'm able to then go through each hypothetical body, system by system if need be, and explain how lifestyle affects them both differently. This simple conceptual comparison allows me to talk about certain aspects of my client's lifestyle and the effects it may have on his or her body, without directly focusing on him or her specifically. In other words, by using made-up people, I'm able to talk about the negative aspects of having an unhealthy body without using my client's body as a constant example. Unhealthy people may get defensive talking about their own bodies, but feel totally comfortable talking about someone else's, especially if they know the person isn't real.

Say I wanted to educate my client on the benefits of cross-training and how it relates to healthy caloric metabolism. The first thing I'd do is introduce them to my two favorite hypothetical people, who just happen to be neighbors, named Zoe and Tanya.

Zoe

Zoe eats a sensible diet, doesn't smoke, and meditates a little every day. (She says it keeps her calm and centered.) On Monday, Wednesday, and Friday she runs or swims for an hour, and on Tuesday and Thursday she works out with free weights at her health club for about the same amount of time. She takes Saturdays off just to relax, and on Sundays she either rides her bike or goes climbing. When there's snow, she substitutes cross-country skiing or aerobics classes for running. She rarely gets sick, and when she does, she recovers quickly. She prides herself on having high energy all day and being able to sleep soundly most nights. She surrounds herself with positive, upbeat, and healthy people because she believes they help her maintain a positive attitude. Zoe is an active, healthy person who just turned forty-three, but looks like a fit thirty-two year old. Her cholesterol level is 165, her resting heart rate is 50 beats per minute and her body fat ratio is 20%.

Tanya

Tanya hasn't exercised in fifteen years (although she recently joined a health club). She smokes (although she's trying to quit) and talks about changing her lifestyle and eating habits, but, "It's hard to find the time." She's been overweight for years, has trouble breathing, and was recently told by her doctor that if she didn't stop smoking and start exercising, she'd be risking a heart attack. She deals with stress by eating chocolate turtles, smoking cigarettes, and making derogatory comments about her boss while having cocktails with coworkers after work.

Tanya goes on a diet for two weeks every year, and once lost fifteen pounds, but gained it back two months later. She always gains back the weight. She inevitably catches whatever cold or flu is going around the office and seems to take forever getting back on her feet. She's lethargic during the day and has trouble sleeping at night. She complains about everything and only seems to lighten up during her after-work cocktails and nachos. Tanya is an inactive, unfit person who just turned forty, and looks much older. Her cholesterol level is 230, her resting heart rate is 90 beats per minute, and her body fat ratio is 33%. Although she feels guilty about it sometimes, she fantasizes about her neighbor Zoe slipping and breaking her leg one morning as she goes out on "her little jog."

After describing both the unhealthy and healthy profiles of Zoe and Tanya, I then take the client on an imaginary 24-hour journey into the bloodstream, muscle cells, and minds of these two women to show how differently their bodies work. **Note:** This educational journey can take as long as you need it to. I have clients, some of whom I've been training for as many as three years, with whom I still use analogies when talking about the benefits of a healthy lifestyle. I find this method of teaching, in conjunction with customized, varied exercise routines, to be the best means of keeping my clients interested in coming back week after week. They are devoted to my exercise program because it offers variety, motivation, continual education, and results.

Now, let's get back to Zoe and Tanya and spend some time snooping around in their bodies.

A Day in the Life

It's six o'clock Monday morning in the town where Zoe and Tanya live. Zoe wakes up refreshed after a great night's sleep, eats breakfast (oatmeal, apple, and orange juice), reads the paper for a half-hour, stretches, and proceeds to go for a morning run. Within the first fifteen minutes of her run, the carbohydrates she ate for breakfast have begun the short journey to be turned into glucose. These glucose molecules are then strung together to form the new glycogen chains her muscle cells will soon be needing to replace the old ones (in storage from last night's dinner) that are beginning to burn up. Ten more minutes into her run, as the new glycogen starts to run low, her liver gets the message to send in the gladiators (fat-burning enzymes). Up to this point, her fat cells have been trickling small amounts of fat into her muscle cells and burning it along with sugar, but as her body senses its glycogen stores getting low, those same fat cells get the signal to open up wide and flood, baby, flood!

As troops of fat-burning enzymes are created and come rushing in to handle the flood, fat quickly takes over as Zoe's main source of fuel. After ten more minutes, pyruvic acid begins to accumulate and her liver is once again called upon, this time to produce the Krebs Cycle enzymes needed to finalize the last stage of fuel-burning. Due to her balanced diet and efficient metabolism, Zoe's liver has no problem creating and maintaining Krebs Cycle enzymes out of the abundance of amino acids that are stored throughout her body.

Zoe lives in the foothills and likes running the trails around her house because they offer a balance of flat and steep terrain. This combination allows her body to remain mostly aerobic and still get the benefit of short spurts of anaerobic exercise. She paces herself for the aerobic part by talking to herself out loud. (She knows that as long as she can talk while running, she's working aerobically and burning fat for fuel.) Her ATP molecules, fed mostly by Krebs Cycle energy, are continually exploded, rebuilt, and exploded again, supplying all the energy her muscles need. If we were to take a peek inside one of Zoe's muscle cells, it would look like a Fourth of July fireworks display with lights flashing, sparks flying, and little explosions happening every second.

Zoe's heart looks like (and is about the size of) a strong muscular fist as it pumps large volumes of oxygenated blood to the far reaches of her capillaries. Enough blood is pumped with each stroke so that it doesn't need to pump as hard or as often as the heart of an unfit person in order to accomplish the same task. This increased stroke volume explains why Zoe's resting heart rate is twenty percent lower than that of the average semi-active person.

Another manifestation of Zoe's strong, efficient heart muscle is lower blood pressure. Over the years, her exercise routine has actually increased the number and size of her capillaries, resulting in less system pressure due to oxygenated blood being dispersed further and with less effort into her muscles. Think of a vein as a garden hose with water flowing through it. Now imagine the pressure that would build up if you were to step on it, compared to letting the same volume of water flow unencumbered through a network of hoses. The pressure would be much less.

Part of the reason Zoe can run trails for an hour and not get winded is that her lungs have become accustomed to saturating her blood with oxygen almost as soon as she breathes it in. Just as her heart doesn't need to pump frantically to distribute blood, her lungs aren't required to respire frantically in order to saturate blood. Because of lower air-intake resistance, her vital capacity (the efficiency with which her lungs expel waste gas) is increased as well as her VO_2 max rating (the rate at which her body absorbs oxygen). Her expanded respiratory passages have increased her breathing capacity to the point that the only time she gets winded is when climbing steep hills. None of the oxygen or nutrients Zoe takes in is wasted. Even at the end of her Krebs Cycle, the leftover water is used to keep her body temperature down through sweating. The other byproduct, carbon dioxide, is mixed with other waste gases and exhaled.

During the hour she's been running, and for at least an hour after, Zoe's mind will remain calm, stress-free, and slightly euphoric due to the fourfold increase in her endorphin levels. These are morphine-like substances that are triggered and released from her pituitary gland whenever she exercises. Although endorphins can be triggered in other ways, such as consuming alcohol, chocolate, tobacco, caffeine, cocaine, etc., the body much prefers producing them through healthier means such as vigorous exercise, sex, pregnancy, or rock climbing. (Hey, I feel them when I climb!)

A fitness research experiment conducted in 1977 at the Baylor College of Medicine by Dr. G. H. Hartung involved comparing forty-eight fit, middle-aged, male runners with an equal number of unfit, middle-aged couch potatoes. At the end of the experiment, Dr. Hartung concluded that the fit group were significantly more intelligent, imaginative, self-sufficient, sober, and calm, and possessed a higher level of well-being than those in the unfit group. Although no direct scientific link has been established between high, naturally-produced endorphin levels and imagination or intelligence, all one need do is talk to an unfit person nursing a hangover, versus a fit person who just ran six miles, and compare what they both have to say. The fit person is likely to exude well-being and seem more intelligent compared with the hung-over guy who may be ready to get sick in front of you.

Tanya's Morning

Tanya's morning didn't go so well. "I'm just not a morning person," she says. She tossed and turned all night and didn't get to sleep until two A.M. Her alarm went off at six, and she promptly smashed it with her fist. Breakfast consisted of two scrambled eggs, three pieces of bacon, a large portion of potatoes, toast with butter, three cups of coffee, two cigarettes, and a diet shake. Within minutes of finishing that last cup of coffee and cigarette, her central nervous system comes raging to life. (Good Morrrrning!) The combination of nicotine and caffeine causes her heart to go into the first of many mild fibrillations she'll experience during the course of her day. (She just sits and waits for them to pass.) Her breathing increases to a rapid pace and her hands tremble slightly as she tries holding the newspaper steady enough to read. After fifteen minutes, the shaking subsides and her heart rate comes back down to her typical 90 beats per minute, allowing her to stand up, go to the bathroom, and take a shower before work.

Tanya's breakfast carbohydrates quickly turn into glucose and proceed to surf her bloodstream looking for muscle cells in need of fuel. After making a few circuits, they realize the futility of their mission and look to her liver for what to do next. Due to her body's sedentary nature, her liver is in no rush to make new glycogen, so it sends this roving glucose off to her fat cells to be stored.

If Tanya does end up having to exert herself somehow during the day, say, by being forced to take the stairs, her blood glucose is depleted so fast that she becomes mildly hypoglycemic, which leads to a big craving for more simple carbohydrates. (This is her body's way of getting her to replace her spent sugar as quickly as possible.) Her body has such a dependence on sugar for fuel that it tries to take in as much as it can, whenever it can, just in case she decides to climb more stairs. The problem is, muscle cells can only store so much sugar, and whatever is left over takes the train to Fat City.

This ties back into the section on insulin and explains the cycle many unfit people get into: overdosing on simple carbohydrates in order to satisfy the hunger that arises after they've depleted their stored glycogen doing minimal anaerobic activity. In the case of an extremely out-of-shape person, something as simple as walking two blocks can deplete blood sugar to the point that he or she will feel faint and need to eat something.

Unfit people tend to spend long periods in a sedentary state, with short sporadic periods of exertion thrown in. Because they may sweat and breathe heavily during sporadic exertion, they may foolishly think they're getting some exercise and burning fat. Ironically, they're only burning sugar and getting fatter. Since they can't burn fat for fuel, their fat cells just get bigger and multiply, while the rest of their system plays sugar catch-up for fuel.

By now, you can see that people like Tanya are in a no-win situation when it comes to caloric metabolism. When Tanya's hyperglycemic after eating too much of the wrong things, her system converts the leftover glucose to fat and stores it. When she's hypoglycemic after doing a short, intense activity, she gets dizzy and hungry and eats more of the wrong things, causing her to become hyperglycemic again, leading to more fat storage. If she dips down into a hypoglycemic state and there is no food to eat, her liver may be forced to take protein and turn it into glucose in order to satisfy her glycogen deficit. This not only causes her muscles to be compromised, but also diminishes her ability to produce important enzymes that could help her to burn fat. (If she'd only exercise!)

The fat in the eggs, bacon, and butter Tanya ate for breakfast has been dumped into her bloodstream, causing it to thicken and move slowly. Some of this fat will surround her organs, some will attach to the walls of her blood vessels, some will be deposited between muscle fibers, and some will become free fatty acids wandering aimlessly in search of active muscles. If no active muscles can be found, these fatty acid molecules retreat to the cushy environment of her fat cells, where they sit dormant and watch TV on little couches that seat three of them together. In order to make more room in fat cells, fatty acids bond together in groups of three called triglycerides. As more and more fatty acids are brought in, the cell gets bigger and ultimately cannot contain all the little couches, so some get booted back out into the bloodstream.

Imagine getting all settled and relaxed on your couch watching TV with two close friends, when BAM! the next minute, you, your friends, and your couch are surfing a tidal wave through the Lincoln Tunnel. (Reminds me of a dream I once had.) If the inside of Zoe's muscle cell looks like a fireworks display, the inside of Tanya's looks like an empty, dimly lit warehouse in the heart of a third-world city. Even robbers don't break in because they know there's nothing to take.

Due to years of physical inactivity, Tanya's liver has all but given up its ability to generate fat-burning enzymes, causing her body to become a huge fat-storage tank surrounded by overtaxed organs and atrophied muscles. Every aspect of her caloric metabolism is utilized for the purpose of burning sugar and storing fat. Unless her lifestyle changes, Tanya will end up dying prematurely of a heart attack or some other preventable disease.

I hope you can see the importance of using this type of creative analogy not only to educate your clients about the benefits of having a healthy lifestyle, but also to get them to take the first step in actually creating one by committing to your fitness program. Since personal trainers generally spend more time with clients than doctors or other health-care professionals, the information we give them about getting and staying fit tends to make a lasting impression.

As I've mentioned before, the primary goal of a successful trainer is to instill in his or her clients a lifetime habit of exercise and health. In my experience, the most important step you can take in achieving this goal is to give your clients a knowledge of how exercise works and to make the application of that knowledge fun. When clients know why your program works and believe that the process can actually be enjoyable, it becomes easier to prove to them, through its application, just how it can change their lives. Be creative and have fun as you point them in this direction. Remember, if you're not having fun teaching your clients about their bodies, they won't have fun learning about them.

*A*fterword

*T*his manual would not be complete without a final word of acknowledgment for you, the personal trainer who wishes to be the best at what you do. No one would question the fact that the guidance and motivation you give people are an integral part of the fitness industry, but a question that sometimes comes up for trainers is this: Are you really worth the money people spend to have you train them?

This is a good question because in reality, people have been exercising for years without the benefit of trainers, and getting results. Why in the last decade has hiring a trainer become so necessary? What is it about this society that encourages certain segments of its population to become so motivated and successful at things like making money, and so unsuccessful at things like staying motivated to exercise and stay fit? In this day and age, shouldn't it be obvious to such people that their health, and the peace of mind it brings, is at least as important as, if not more important than, their careers, what kind of cars they drive, or how much money they can make?

The answer is: Of course it should! But after many years of personal training, I've come to realize that for a lot of folks, it's not. Not that I'm trying to diminish the importance of having a successful career, but when that becomes the main focus of a person's life, it is often at the expense of his or her health and well-being. The shortsighted priorities that some people establish for their lives continually baffle me.

However, for those people who have come to realize that a balance is in order, you and I become a valuable resource. Why? Because good personal trainers help to establish health as a priority in people's lives. They help people to balance career success with good health, and this is the primary reason they are willing to pay us what we charge. It is worth it to them to maintain a more balanced perspective, and that becomes the core of our service.

The reason I'm so obsessed with our service being the best it can be (and the main reason I wrote this book) is that I have a personal stake in this whole thing. This industry is important to me because it provides not only my livelihood, but also the livelihood of some four hundred thousand other hardworking trainers across the country. Call me selfish, or self-serving, but the bottom line is, if you choose to make personal training a career and do the job poorly, it makes the whole industry look bad. And if the industry looks bad, I, and every other serious trainer in the country, have to work that much harder to make it look good.

Obviously, you bought and read this book because you are one of those trainers who are striving to make our industry shine. You understand the importance of being the best, even though you may never experience the glamour or recognition of training movie celebrities, high-ranking politicians, rock stars, or Navy SEALS. You strive to excel at personal training, in spite of the fact that you may never have your own early morning cable TV show filmed on the sunny beaches of Hawaii or Malibu. You'll most likely be found working in regular health clubs or in your own fitness studio, training busy soccer moms, store managers, teachers, doctors, stockbrokers, and realtors. You subscribe to a realistic and functional approach to exercise and try hard to stay knowledgeable, motivated, and patient. At some point in your life, you became aware that you were actually good at motivating others to do healthy things and decided to make a career of it. What could be more honorable and rewarding than using this talent to guide people to longer, healthier, more productive lives through the use of your exercise program and a proper diet?

In response to those who ask if you are really worth the amount of money you charge for your services, I have this question: What could be more valuable than helping people to establish lifetime habits of health through the mentality of prevention and physical activity? I can't think of anything.

In closing, I'd like to leave you with this final thought: It really does take more than just making people sweat to get them to change from an unhealthy lifestyle to a healthy one. Sometimes it takes a lot of guidance and the heart of a great personal trainer. I am honored to have the opportunity to work with you to bring these changes to pass. Thank you for taking the time to read my book. See you at the gym!

Books Available From Robert D. Reed Publishers

Please include payment with orders. Send indicated book/s to:

Name:_____

Address:_____

City:_____ State:_____ Zip:_____

Phone:(____)_____ E-mail:_____

Titles and Authors	Unit Price
It's More Than Just Making Them Sweat by Ed Thornton	$11.95
Gotta Minute? The ABC's of Successful Living by Tom Massey, Ph.D., N.D.	9.95
Gotta Minute? Practical Tips for Abundant Living: The ABC's of Total Health by Tom Massey, Ph.D., N.D.	9.95
Gotta Minute? How to Look & Feel Great! by Marcia F. Kamph, M.S., D.C.	11.95
Gotta Minute? Yoga for Health, Relaxation & Well-being by Nirvair Singh Khalsa	9.95
Gotta Minute? Ultimate Guide of One-Minute Workouts for Anyone, Anywhere, Anytime! by Bonnie Nygard, M.Ed. & Bonnie Hopper, M.Ed.	9.95
A Kid's Herb Book For Children Of All Ages by Lesley Tierra, Acupuncturist and Herbalist	19.95
House Calls: How we can all heal the world one visit at a time by Patch Adams, M.D.	11.95
500 Tips For Coping With Chronic Illness by Pamela D. Jacobs, M.A.	11.95

Enclose a copy of this order form with payment for books. Send to the address below. Shipping & handling: $2.50 for first book plus $1.00 for each additional book. California residents add 8.5% sales tax. We offer discounts for large orders.

Please make checks payable to: Robert D. Reed Publishers.
Total enclosed: $_____. See our website for more books!

Robert D. Reed Publishers
750 La Playa, Suite 647, San Francisco, CA 94121
Phone: 650-994-6570 • Fax: 650-994-6579
Email: 4bobreed@msn.com • www.rdrpublishers.com